THE EssentialYoga
PROGRAM

CREATING MONTHLY WORKSHOPS
INTRODUCING dōTERRA®
ESSENTIAL OILS

Library of Congress Control Number: 2014904325

ISBN 978-0-9916407-0-6

Design: Huddleston Marketing & Design
Editing: Bettina Moench

Version 2

We dedicate this guidebook to the founders of
dōTERRA, who had the vision, courage and talent
to bring these amazing gifts of the earth into
our lives. Love you guys and gal!

We also want to thank our instructors and guides,
families and friends and our dōTERRA team members...
all of whose support and encouragement to

dream a little bigger,

stretch a little further,

breathe a little deeper and

reach a little higher

has made this possible.

Namasté,

Jane, Marty, Deidra and Stephanie

*NAMASTÉ: I honor the place in you in which the entire universe dwells. I honor
the place in you which is of love, of truth, of light and of peace. When you
are in that place in you, and I am in that place in me, we are one.*

Envisioning The EssentialYoga Program

The EssentialYoga Program is the result of a collaboration that brings together our varied yet similar paths and our shared love of both dōTERRA® essential oils and yoga. Yoga transforms our physical, emotional and spiritual lives while essential oils have been used throughout history to support and heal those same connections. This book reflects our dedication to uniting these two complementary practices.

The EssentialYoga Program stems from our diverse experiences and backgrounds as yoga instructors, students and oil enthusiasts. We realized that essential oils are a beautiful complement to any yoga practice and began creating monthly workshops integrating oils and yoga. The workshops were consistently a great success, where we witnessed students excited about the powerful impact and nurturing quality the oils had on their yoga practice. At the same time, interest emerged outside the studio from those who wanted to share dōTERRA oils as a complementary therapy with their yoga friends.

This inspired us to create The EssentialYoga Program with 12 months of our favorite workshops for the yoga studio owner, teacher, student and curious bystander who loves oils! We are passionate about incorporating dōTERRA's CPTG Certified Pure Therapeutic Grade® oils into our personal well-being and sharing these oils with our students and friends. In doing so, we have favorably impacted yoga practitioners around the world while enjoying the opportunity to create financial abundance for many.

It is our intention that The EssentialYoga Program afford you the same creativity, fun and success in your yoga practice and teachings that we have enjoyed in creating its content. We enthusiastically present dōTERRA essential oils to the yoga community as a powerful way to enhance the practice, teachings and business of yoga.

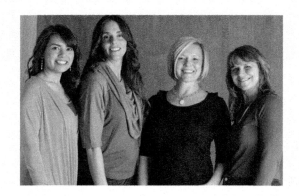

Deidra Schaub, Jane Bloom,
Stephanie Smith and Marty Harger
Co-creators of The EssentialYoga Program

Table of Contents

"The earth is our mother. Whatever befalls the earth befalls the sons and daughters of the earth. This we know.

All things are connected like the blood which unites one family. All things are connected. We did not weave the web of life, we are merely strands in it. Whatever we do to the web we do to ourselves."

—CHIEF SEATTLE

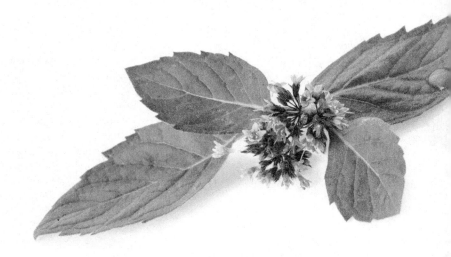

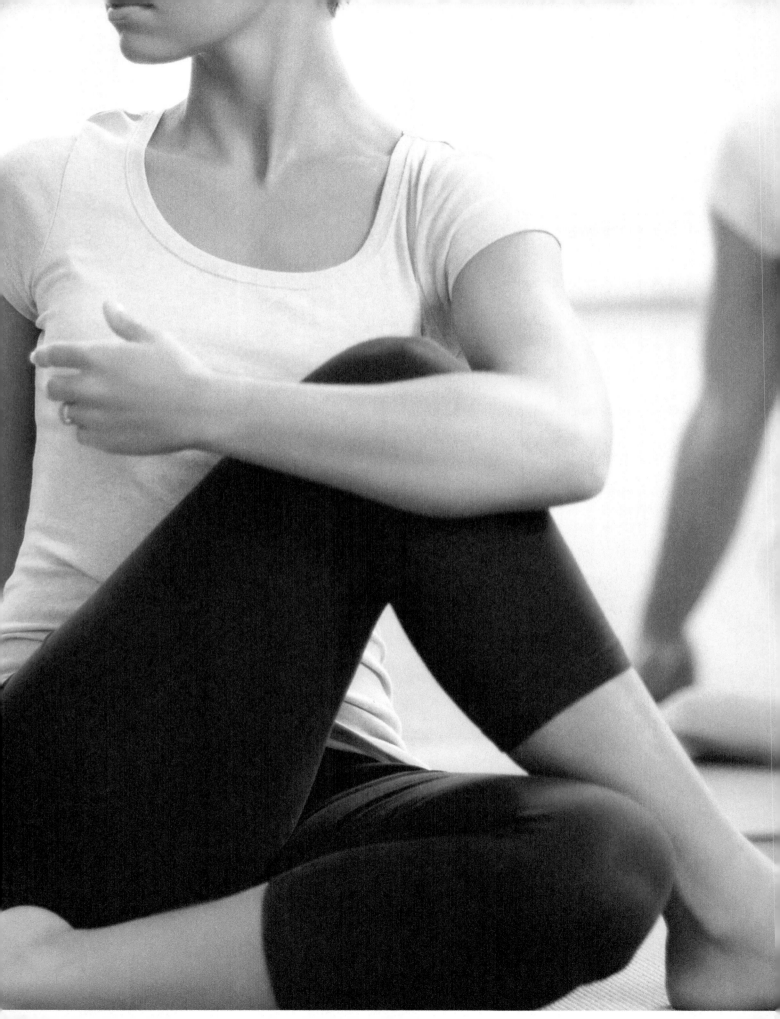

Welcome to
The EssentialYoga Program

We are excited to present this guide to empower you and your yoga students with new and creative choices using dōTERRA essential oils to help improve your practice, health and well-being.

The EssentialYoga Program combines our experience teaching yoga and enhancing our own health and businesses with dōTERRA essential oils. Although the Program is written as a guidebook for yoga instructors and studio owners, **anyone wanting to combine their interests and passion for yoga and essential oils** will enjoy the material we've developed. Throughout this guidebook you'll see ideas to make the exploration of dōTERRA essential oils with yoga a fun experience for you and your students. We've offered direction, alternative options and the flexibility to make these workshops your own. Our ideas run the spectrum from the simplest ways to include the essential oils in your classes and business, to a complete and detailed annual curriculum of themed, monthly workshops you can offer in your studio or bring to a place you choose to teach, to extensive dōTERRA business-building tips.

Expanding Your Practice

Yoga instructors and studio owners often are asked for advice and suggestions on holistic health choices. Essential oils from dōTERRA are a great recommendation for your students, as they are an excellent addition to any natural and healthy lifestyle. In this guidebook we'll suggest sources you can turn to for further knowledge on essential oils and their use for your personal health.

Weaving essential oils into your yoga practice can deepen and expand your yoga experience in new dimensions with just a few powerful, healing drops. Essential oils, like yoga, are both simple and complex. A single oil or blend can be used for a specific intended purpose, yet that same oil or blend also can address multiple aspects of healing the body, mind and spirit.

Over time as you incorporate dōTERRA essential oils into your life and yoga practice, you will get to know the way they work with your body and mind. You will come to learn and sense which oils can help you calm, energize and lift mood, take in your deepest breath, and connect you with your innermost thoughts. The knowledge provided in this book, along with other resources suggested, will guide you in sharing the oils with your students.

Bringing Nature into the Studio

Yoga allows us the time to tune out the world and go within. Studios strive to create a natural environment free of distraction for students. Decor, lighting and music each affect the ability to focus on one's own practice that day. When we add the natural, harmonizing earth element of plants into our practice space through the use and application of essential oils, we enhance the experience by bringing in the unique aroma and powerful healing energy each plant provides. Essential oils assist us in balancing our body, mind and spirit, helping us to recognize the beautiful peace that surrounds and supports us in each moment if we will take the time to "smell the roses."

Why Use dōTERRA Essential Oils?

These natural, therapeutic aromatic compounds are provided by a company called dōTERRA, whose name means "Gift of the Earth." dōTERRA's rapid rise to become the world's leading essential oil company is no surprise once you open a bottle of their CPTG Certified Pure Therapeutic Grade essential oils and inhale their crisp and clean aromas. But once you begin using their oils aromatically, topically and even internally, you'll begin to truly discover their therapeutic difference.

dōTERRA searches the world for the highest quality source of each oil and blend they offer, and then conducts rigorous scientific tests to ensure their quality. The EssentialYoga Program evolved from our relationships with these powerful healing tools that, simply put, have no equal in the world of essential oils. The EssentialYoga Program would never have been created if we hadn't met dōTERRA, and therefore, each other.

The Powerful Synergy of Yoga and Essential Oils

Adding essential oils to the yoga practice accelerates or enhances the student's ability to overcome the mind through the body. Historically, oils have been used to aid in meditation that brings us to the present moment. By combining oils and yoga, we bring the two disciplines together to heighten the impact for the student. The EssentialYoga Program and workshop suggestions uniquely offer the benefit of extending the impact or influence of the yoga practice beyond the mat. In our monthly workshop approach, students will experience the immediate effects of the oils. Those who then choose to purchase dōTERRA oils for their personal home use will recognize the extended health value from your EssentialYoga workshop.

Why "Workshop" with Oils?

Introducing The EssentialYoga Program to your students and studio creates a truly special event. **This is NOT your everyday yoga class!** It is something NEW and exciting, and thus we've titled our program as such – a "workshop." The workshops outlined in this guidebook will typically take 90 minutes to teach with an additional 1/2 hour for questions afterward. If you'd like some help learning more about the oils or leading your workshop, ask the person who introduced you to dōTERRA to join you in launching this exciting new series at your studio. It's a wonderful way to combine efforts for even better results.

The oils work differently on every body, and you and your students may find yourselves drawn to different oils at different times. What better "gift" can we give to one another than the gift of choice? This is our gift to you in The EssentialYoga Program. We believe that empowering you to choose how *you* use the oils and share them is the greatest gift of all. In our Program, we encourage you take our suggestions and adapt them to your needs. We have even included information on how to pay for your oils or supplement your income.

Empowering You to Choose

Our Program is a guideline and intended to give you ideas to customize your own practice, classes, business and life. We each know our body, mind and spirit best. dōTERRA teaches us to become our own oil expert and experiment with the oils as we apply them aromatically, topically and internally. As The EssentialYoga Program's creators, we are so grateful and honored to be able to use and share these beautiful plant essences from all over the world in our daily lives. They have made all the difference for each of us in our own way. By empowering ourselves to make healthier, natural choices, we offer the same to you.

It is in the spirit of empowering you with choices, that we have created The EssentialYoga Program.

EssentialYoga Workshops Are for Everyone

The EssentialYoga Program workshops are adaptable to suit a variety of yoga experiences and abilities. This is a means to increase, expand and deepen one's practice. Enjoy offering our workshops for all forms of hatha yoga.

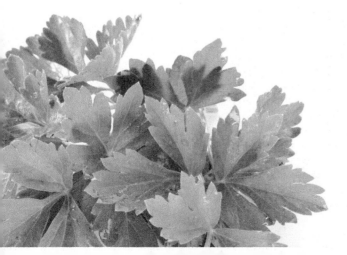

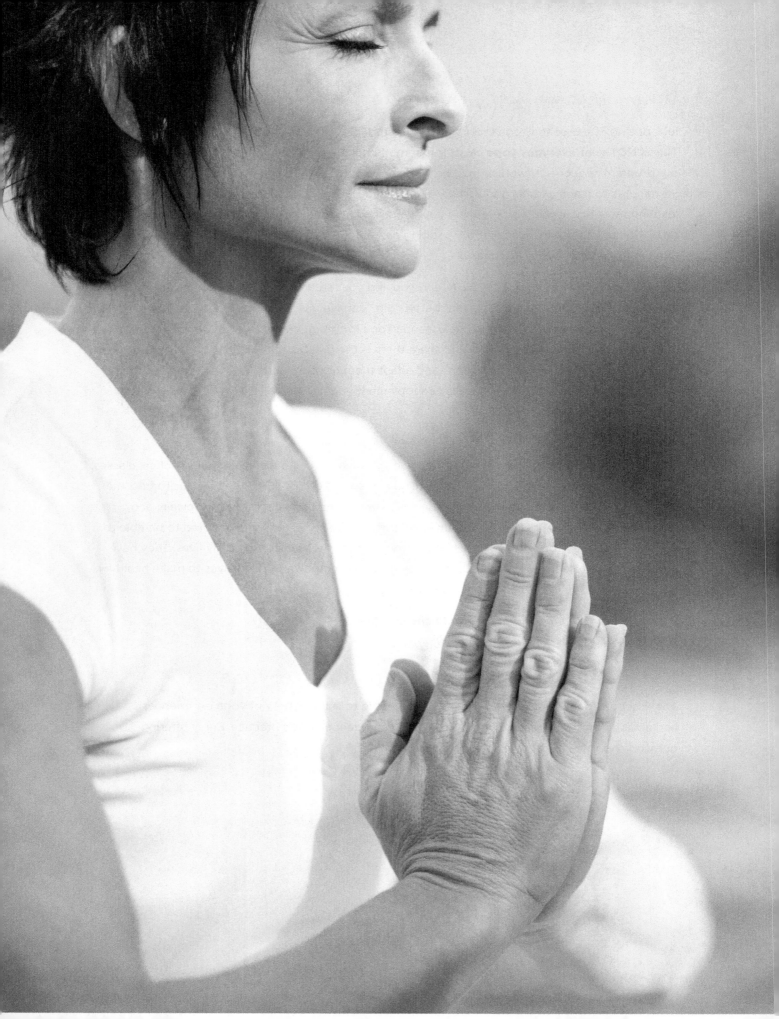

Essential Oils and Yoga

Oils Throughout History

Essential oils have been used for therapeutic and spiritual purposes for thousands of years. Plants were grown and harvested for their medicinal and aromatic properties. Both dried herbs and oils were created and used in many forms – aromatically, topically and internally. Early historic records show extensive use of essential oils in the Egyptian culture, as well as in Mesopotamia, India and China. They are referenced in all major religious scriptures for physical, meditative and spiritual purposes. Distillation processes were developed over time to extract the essential oil from the raw plant material. Interestingly, most essential oils are still produced at small family farms around the world, using the extraction method that has been used for over 3,000 years. A valued commodity for their medicinal, healing traits, essential oils were exchanged or traded as a form of commerce in many cultures. According to the World Health Organization (WHO), it is estimated that 80% of the world's population currently uses herbal medicine for some aspect of primary health care[1].

The use of essential oils to enhance and complement the yoga practice dates back thousands of years and originated in India with **sandalwood** and **vetiver.** Essential oils are a component of the holistic Ayurvedic view that addresses dosha imbalances of heating and cooling, moisture and dryness. There are many wonderful reference books for those interested in a personalized selection of essential oils for dosha balancing, which we have listed in the Appendix. For the purposes of The EssentialYoga Program, we focus on the historic connection between two aspects of traditional Ayurvedic practice: yoga and essential oils.

Yoga and Ayurveda are two interrelated healing disciplines originating in India under the Vedic system. Ayurveda addresses all aspects of healing and well-being for body and mind. "Yoga… outlines the prime principles and methods for developing the meditative mind that is the basis of all Vedic knowledge," according to author and Ayurvedic expert David Frawley.

"Ayurveda is one of the world's oldest holistic (whole-body) healing systems. It developed thousands of years ago in India. It is based on the belief that health and wellness depend on a delicate balance between the mind, body, and spirit. The primary focus of Ayurvedic medicine is to promote good health, rather than fight disease. But treatments may be recommended for specific health problems."[2]

Aromatherapy and Our Sense of Scent

There is significant research on our sense of scent through the field of aromatherapy. For instance, the human nose is said to be able to detect nearly 10,000 unique aromas – each eliciting a psychological response – favorable or unfavorable[3]. This innate skill helped ancient hunter-gatherers to sense danger or attraction and health or illness in one another and their surroundings.

Aromas stay with us. In fact, one year after inhaling a scent, studies have shown that people are able to recall it with 65% accuracy. Think about how that retained sense of smell will favorably affect a yoga student's ability to go within and recreate sensations experienced in your EssentialYoga workshop or to remember your studio.

Although not a common concern, not everyone can detect aroma. Anosmia is the name for the partial or complete lack of ability to smell that usually comes as a result of head injury, infection or blockage of the nose. Some medications and even mood can diminish or enhance our ability to detect aroma.

Regardless of one's ability to detect unique aromas in your workshop, essential oils are so much more than a pretty scent – **they are therapeutically powerful** and when applied to the skin or inhaled aromatically through the nose, their chemistry creates a beneficial impact on everyone in the studio. For those sensitive to aroma, it is best to direct them to other yoga workshops more appropriate than one using essential oils, as any EssentialYoga Program workshop will include enhanced use of oils and may create adverse effects for their particular sensitivity. In our experience, however, even those with allergies rarely develop unfavorable reactions to the dōTERRA oils, primarily because of their purity and because sensitivity often is to pollen, not aroma.

Accelerate the Relaxation Effect with Essential Oils

In our EssentialYoga workshops, we create a "scent memory" for the student – helping them connect to the breath and recall the moment of presence they experienced on their yoga mat. Aroma connects directly to our parasympathetic nervous system – the branch of the autonomic nervous system that controls the peripheral organs and the ability to remain calm and relaxed. Inhaling aromas reaches the emotional aspect of our subconscious quickly – which is why our sense of scent is such a powerful emotional healing tool. Think how aromas tap into your memory bank – the smell of fresh-baked pie reminds you of picking apples with your beloved grandmother, or roasted peanuts send you back to your first trip to the zoo. With any yoga practice, we tap into the parasympathetic nervous system and the body's natural relaxation response. **The use of essential oils accelerates the relaxation effect in the workshop, helps reduce stress and thus supports healthy immune function.**

Add Essential Oils To Your Practice

Essential oils provide a true vibrational healing tool. They subtly complement the yoga practice as they affect the mood and emotion on a conscious and subconscious level.

Learn more about the therapeutic health advantages you, your family, students and the world can experience by even the simplest choices these fast-acting, cost-effective and natural plant remedies offer. Turn to one of the suggested resources in the Appendix for excellent reference books and trusted websites to learn more about essential oils.

TIP | Diffusing essential oils in your studio, home or office is a perfect way to help relieve tension, dispel odors and create an atmosphere of peace and harmony. Diffusing essential oils has been reported to support the immune system and create a feeling of balance and well-being.

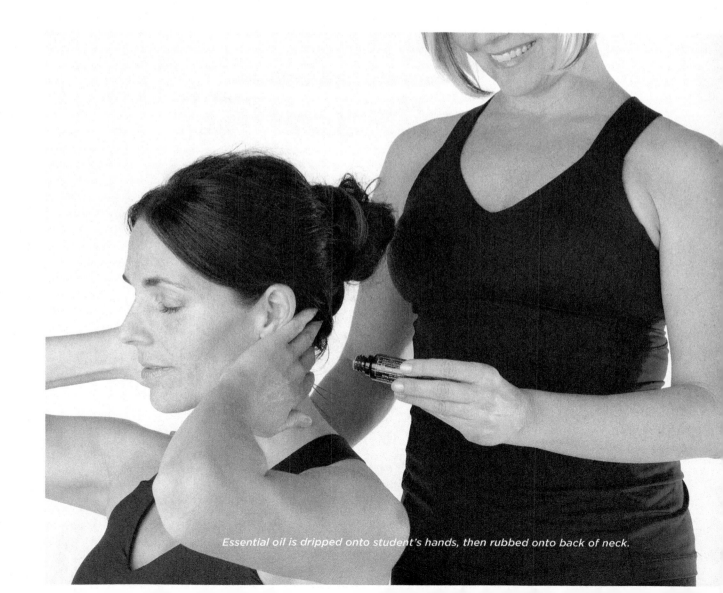

Essential oil is dripped onto student's hands, then rubbed onto back of neck.

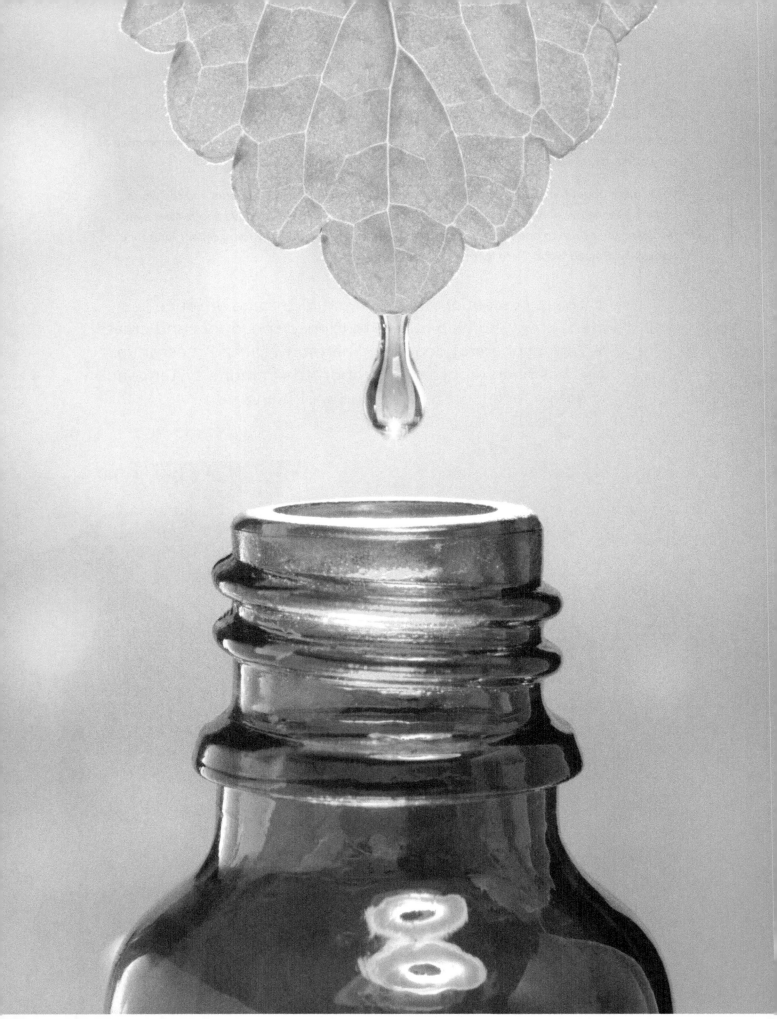

Recommended Oil Source and Use

Essential oils are highly concentrated, aromatic, liquid plant essences. The oils originate primarily from herbs, flowers and trees and are contained in the seeds, bark, roots, resin, flower petals, rind and leaves. The dōTERRA essential oils we suggest are generally extracted from the plant substance via steam distillation, although cold expression is used for citrus oils. They can be both beautifully and powerfully fragrant, eliciting profound emotional responses. Yet the use of essential oils goes well beyond their fragrant appeal. Used throughout history for their medicinal and therapeutic benefits, essential oils can be used as natural alternatives in holistic self-care practices. Their unique chemistry allows them to be used aromatically and applied topically to the skin, while other essential oils can be used as dietary aids to promote vitality and well-being. To create even a drop of essential oil often requires hundreds of pounds of plant material. Treat them as the "gifts of the earth" they are, and be conscious of the amount you use at a time, as often just two or three drops will do. No matter how you use the oils – aromatically, topically, internally – they will work their magic and go to work on those around them.

 TIP It can be very powerful to incorporate essential oils into mantra and/or meditation work. You will feel the vibration of the entire room rise.

Why dōTERRA Essential Oils?

dōTERRA® (meaning "Gift of the Earth") essential oils represent the safest, purest essential oils available in the world today. Each of the dōTERRA CPTG Certified Pure Therapeutic Grade® essential oils is carefully extracted by a global network of skilled growers, distillers and chemists, ensuring a consistently powerful user experience. They are pure aromatic extracts, contain no artificial ingredients and are tested to be free of contaminants, such as pesticides or other chemical residues.

The authors of The EssentialYoga Program have used a variety of essential oil brands for years. For each of us, our introduction to dōTERRA's pure, clean, crisp scents was only the beginning of a complete transformation from other oils, to exclusive use of dōTERRA oils, blends and products. Why? If you haven't already experienced the dōTERRA difference, see the person who shared The EssentialYoga Program with you, or contact one of us. It starts with aroma, but honestly, the true commitment to dōTERRA-only lifestyles, yoga workshops and businesses came as a result of the profound physiologic and emotional healing responses we each have had with dōTERRA oils. **dōTERRA oils are simply the highest quality essential oils in the world!**

dōTERRA's Company Vision and Mission Is Clear

When using or teaching The EssentialYoga Program, we believe it is important to understand the values, vision and mission of the company that provides dōTERRA essential oils. Please take a minute to read the following.

"We at dōTERRA are committed to sharing the life-enhancing benefits of therapeutic-grade essential oils and essential oil enhanced wellness products with the world. We will do this by:

• Discovering and developing the world's highest-quality, therapeutic-grade essential oil products through a leveraged network of highly educated and experienced botanists, chemists, health scientists and health-care professionals.

• Producing our essential oil products to the highest standard of quality, purity and safety used in the industry—CPTG Certified Pure Therapeutic Grade®.

• Distributing our products through Wellness Advocates who, working from home, introduce, educate, and sell dōTERRA® wellness products locally through person-to-person contact and globally through personalized web shopping sites.

• Providing educational opportunities for all people interested in learning how therapeutic-grade essential oils can be used as a self-care wellness alternative.

• Bringing together health-care professionals of traditional and alternative medicine to encourage further study and application of therapeutic-grade essential oils in modern health-care practices."

The dōTERRA Difference?

CPTG Certified Pure Therapeutic Grade®

THE FOLLOWING INFORMATION THROUGH PAGE 18 ON DŌTERRA'S QUALITY CONTROL PROCESS IS PROVIDED BY DŌTERRA INTERNATIONAL, LLC.

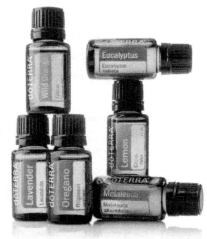

dōTERRA CPTG Certified Pure Therapeutic Grade* essential oils are pure, natural aromatic compounds carefully extracted from plants. They do not contain fillers or artificial ingredients that would dilute their active qualities. Proper extraction and quality control methods also ensure that dōTERRA essential oils are free of any contaminants such as pesticides or other chemical residues.

In addition to being pure and natural, dōTERRA essential oils are subjected to additional quality testing that ensures the correct composition of the active natural compounds found in each oil.

Even though an essential oil may be pure, if the right species or part of a plant has not been used, or if the plant has not been grown in the right environment or harvested at the right time, or if it has not been distilled under the right conditions, the natural chemical makeup of the extraction will not provide as predictable and powerful a benefit. In some cases, the wrong plant harvested at the wrong time may result in an extract that contains harmful levels of some constituents.

dōTERRA essential oils are guaranteed to be pure, natural and free of synthetic compounds or contaminates. They are subjected to rigorous Mass Spectrometry and Gas Chromatography testing to ensure extract composition and activity. dōTERRA pure essential oils represent the safest and most beneficial essential oils available today.

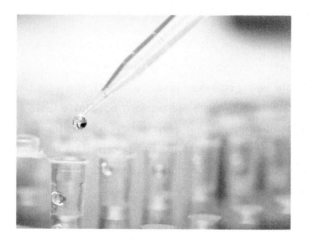

Equally stringent standards of safety and efficacy are applied to all of the dōTERRA Essential Wellness products. Guided by the Scientific Advisory Board and Health-Care Professional Committee, dōTERRA uses only top development and manufacturing partners who maintain GMP certification and enjoy industry reputation for superior innovation and quality work product. Each dōTERRA product is guaranteed to exceed customer satisfaction for quality and efficacy.

CPTG Testing Methods
Quality Control for dōTERRA Essential Oils

dōTERRA's CPTG Certified Pure Therapeutic Grade* quality protocol employs five different analytical methods to ensure dōTERRA's essential oils are both pure (extracts have only the volatile aromatic compounds of a plant), and potent (have consistent chemical composition from batch to batch). The CPTG quality protocol requires the use of independent laboratories for standardization and testing.

Test 1: Gas Chromatography

After the aromatic compounds (also called essential oils) are carefully distilled from plant material, samples are tested for chemical composition using gas chromatography. In gas chromatography, volatile essential oil compounds are vaporized and passed through a long column called a gas chromatograph. Each individual compound travels or "elutes" through the column at a different

---

CPTG Certified Pure Therapeutic Grade is a registered trademark of dōTERRA Holdings, LLC representing internal standards of quality assessment and material control. The CPTG testing protocols require the use of independent laboratories for CPTG standardization and quality testing. The CPTG protocol is not administered by government or industry regulatory agencies and does not imply regulatory approval of dōTERRA protocols.

rate and is measured as it exits the column during the testing period. Using gas chromatography, quality control engineers can determine which compounds are present in a test sample and, as importantly, at what levels.

Test 2: Mass Spectrometry

In addition to gas chromatography, essential oil samples also are tested for composition using mass spectrometry. In mass spectrometry, samples are vaporized and then ionized and each individual compound in a sample is measured by weight. Mass spectrometry provides additional insight to the purity of an essential oil by revealing the presence of non-aromatic compounds, such as heavy metals or other pollutants, which are too heavy to elute along a gas chromatograph. The combination of gas chromatography and mass spectrometry is sometimes referred to as a GC/MS test.

Test 3: FTIR Scan *(Fourier Transform Infrared Spectroscopy)*

After an essential oil passes the gas chromatography and mass spectrometry tests, it is transported to a manufacturing facility for filling. Before being released into the facility, the essential oil "batch" is held in quarantine while additional quality tests are performed. Those tests include a FTIR Scan, which, similar to GC/MS testing, is also an analysis of material composition. In a FTIR Scan, a light is shown at the material sample and the amount of light absorbed by the chemical constituents of the sample is measured. Results are then compared against an historical database to ensure adherence to composition standards.

Test 4: Microbial Testing

Before a batch of essential oils can be released from quarantine to manufacturing, it must be tested for the presence of bio-hazards such as bacteria, fungus, and mold. In microbial testing, samples are drawn from each batch of essential oils and applied to growing mediums in dishes or "plates." After an incubation period, each plate is analyzed for growth of microbes. This test is performed on all incoming material to the manufacturing facility, and also performed on finished product to ensure no harmful organisms have been introduced to the product during the filling and labeling process, and to ensure shelf-life stability.

Test 5: Organoleptic Testing

Organoleptic testing brings a human touch to each step of the CPTG quality control process. Organoleptics include those attributes of an essential oil that can be tested with taste, sight, touch and smell. From growers and harvesters to essential oil chemists; from manufacturing engineers to essential oil practitioners; dōTERRA's global network of essential oil providers carefully monitors the quality of each CPTG Certified Pure Therapeutic Grade essential oil. The extraction of essential oils is very much an art form that can be enhanced by, but not replaced with, mechanical analytics. The wisdom and experience of dōTERRA's essential oil experts are an indispensable part of the CPTG quality control standard.

Three Ways to Effectively Use dōTERRA Essential Oils

1. Aromatic Application

The field of aromatherapy is the common term for the aromatic diffusion of essential oils to create a therapeutic impact. Many research studies have directly tied the impact on mood and emotion that essential oil diffusion can create. Oils can simply be dropped on the hands, rubbed together and cupped around the nose. They can be added to distilled water in a spray bottle and misted around the room or on a person. Drops can be placed in a diffuser to disperse a mist into the air and create an aromatic and therapeutic "bubble" around those in a room that they will inhale for benefit.

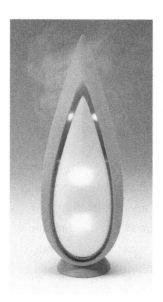

One of our favorite dōTERRA essential oil diffusers is the **Lotus diffuser** because of its special air pump designed to disperse essential oils in a micro-fine mist that stays suspended for several hours. Diffused oils don't just mask odors; they actually alter the structure of the molecules that create odors and eliminate them. Diffusing releases oxygenating molecules as well as negative ions, which kill microbes. Research shows that cold-air diffusing certain essential oils may:

- Reduce unpleasant odors
- Relax the mind and body, relieve tension and clear the mind
- Help with weight management
- Improve concentration, alertness and mental clarity

Before you begin your workshop, ask students about any known plant sensitivities and avoid application to that individual.

2. Topical Application

We apply oils topically to have a therapeutic effect on a part or all of the body. We often think of topical application for physical needs, but as we apply the oils on our skin, we also take in the aromatic benefits. For instance, applying **peppermint** essential oil to the chest opens respiration, and the aroma also stimulates the mind and uplifts the heart. The adaptogenic nature of essential oils allows our bodies to take in what we need, and use it to bring balance to our being. Remarkably, essential oils can affect every cell of the body in just 20 minutes![4]

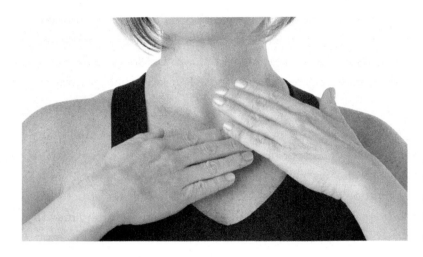

Applying essential oils to the chest benefits the cells of the body and provides a wonderful aromatic impact during your yoga practice.

When applying essential oils topically, many people first dilute them using a "carrier" vegetable oil, butter or wax. Carrier oils are plant-based, but don't have the concentrated aroma or therapeutic value of essential oils. Their role is to dilute essential oils or carry them over a larger area of skin. Common choices for carrier oils include **Fractionated Coconut Oil** (fat has been removed to allow an unscented/non-staining liquid carrier that is great for use with dōTERRA essential oils), and cold-pressed oils such as sesame, olive, almond, grapeseed, avocado, walnut and many others.

Less is more with essential oils! In EssentialYoga workshops, you will be using just a small amount per student when applying oils during the workshop. Remember, these are highly concentrated plant essences. You only need two to three drops of dōTERRA essential oils every two to three hours to have a therapeutic effect topically. You can dilute those drops into a carrier to spread the oil or blend across more of the body's surface, or you can apply some of the oils "neat," or undiluted. dōTERRA essential oils are clearly labeled to indicate which oils are suggested for dilution or can be applied neat without concern, and which are intended for internal as well as topical and aromatic use.

The oils will have the same impact on the body whether diluted or undiluted, and will usually take effect within just a few minutes of application. Essential oils are lipophilic – meaning they can penetrate the outer membrane of the body's fat cells, and move directly into the lymphatic and circulatory systems below the surface of the skin. From the skin's surface, these systems transport the essential oils and their therapeutic chemical constituents throughout the body and toward areas where their presence will assist in creating balance when imbalance exists.

One important note: We often apply essential oils to the bottoms of the feet. Why the feet? In the study of reflexology (sometimes referred to as Zoneology or reflex therapy) essential oils are applied to the bottom of the foot on specific points relating to body organs, systems and nerve pathways. Our feet are one of the most nerve-rich parts of the body, with thousands of nerve endings per foot. As the oils are applied and massaged into the foot's pores and many sweat glands, the body pulls the oils in and puts them to work.

3. Internal Application

dōTERRA's Certified Pure Therapeutic Grade Essential Oils are safe for internal use, due to the rigorous testing the company performs on EVERY batch of oils, EVERY time (see CPTG Certified Pure Therapeutic Grade Testing Methods section). However, not every oil brand is appropriate for internal consumption (see bottle label for Supplement Facts if appropriate to consume). In The EssentialYoga Program, we suggest some specific oils you can try for internal use, such as citrus oils and other oils commonly used as spices or flavorings in cooking such as **cassia, ginger, peppermint** and **spearmint.** Add two to three drops to 32 ounces of water, shake and pour a sample for workshop attendees.

Internal use of dōTERRA essential oils is suggested to assist in supporting digestive and immune health, for flavoring and for oral hygiene. This method is NOT recommended with any other brand of essential oils.

If you are not comfortable with the internal approach, aromatic
and topical alternative application is also effective!

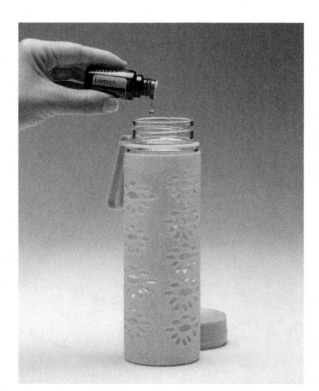

Always use a glass, ceramic or stainless steel container when mixing dōTERRA oils into water or other liquids.

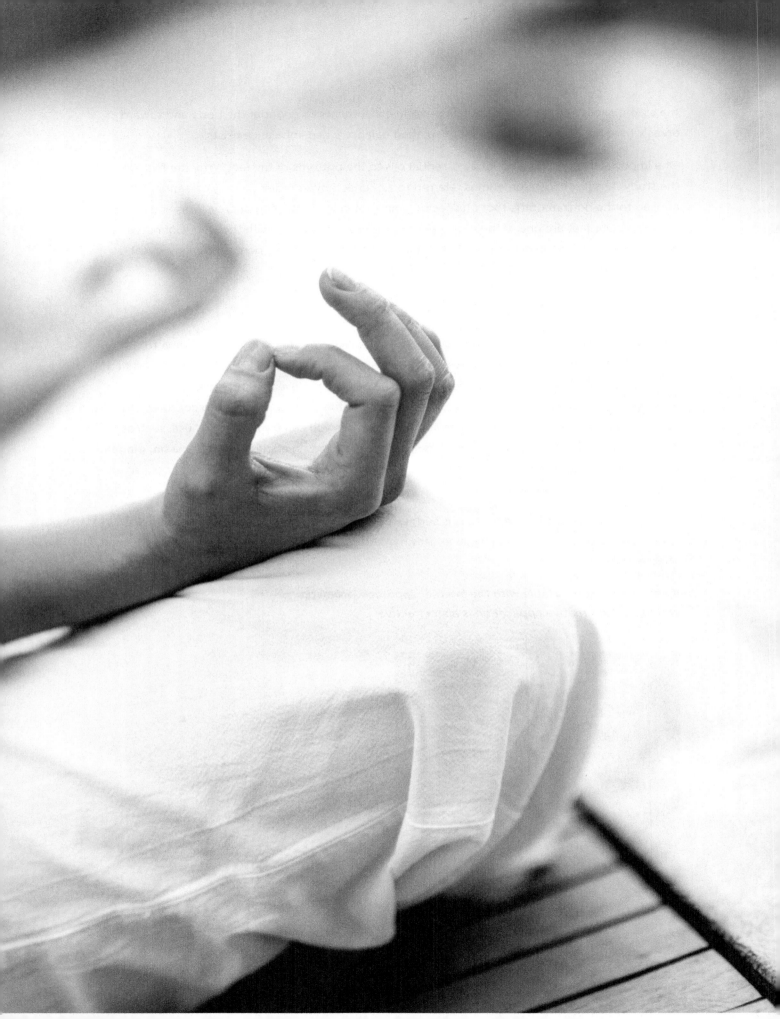

Twelve Months of EssentialYoga

"The mind lives in the past and the future; the oils bring you back to the present."

– JERI MCDOWELL
Certified Yoga Instructor

The EssentialYoga Program's calendar of workshops was designed with ease and choice in mind. Workshop planning has been simplified with this go-to monthly reference guide, providing yoga practitioners and instructors the knowledge and steps to confidently integrate six to seven essential oils into a theme-based monthly EssentialYoga Workshop.

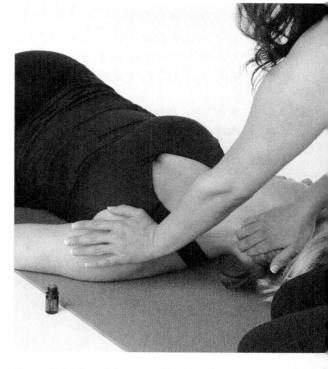

Essential oils add a new dimension, creating a relaxing and comforting connection in the workshop setting.

• Each workshop is designed with a monthly themed sequence that includes the suggested dōTERRA essential oils.

• Specific oils were chosen to enhance the physical and emotional aspects of the workshop.

• Monthly outlines offer a theme that works effectively with any discipline or tradition of yoga.

• Suggested hatha yoga postures also are offered for a sequencing template that can be followed as is or modified into a yoga style of your choice.

• It is highly recommended to have one assistant per six-to-eight students to aid in oil application.

• For your convenience, both retail and wholesale dōTERRA essential oil cost information is provided as a guideline on the price you may wish to charge for your workshop. See dōTERRA Essential Oil Pricing section for more ideas.

• Instructor note: Single-side sequences are to be repeated on the opposite side.

dōTERRA Essential Oils will infuse and enhance the yoga practitioner's experience through aroma, topical application and internal use. The oils and type of application are paired with specific yoga poses to facilitate an experience centered on a theme and physical or energetic focus. For example, during beginning breathwork the instructor may use **frankincense** oil, which has been used in meditative practice for centuries to promote grounding and focus. Later, the **Balance blend** oil may be applied to the feet prior to a balancing sequence.

EssentialYoga workshops are approximately 90 minutes in length, although **many studios prefer to leave two full hours for the workshops** to allow for discussion afterwards. Workshops are broken down into specific segments, which are delineated in the workshop template and explained in greater detail in the workshop script. On the following pages is a detailed workshop preparation list and sample script to better familiarize you with the content meant to be shared throughout a workshop. Please note that the sample script on the following pages is denoted by the words in blue.

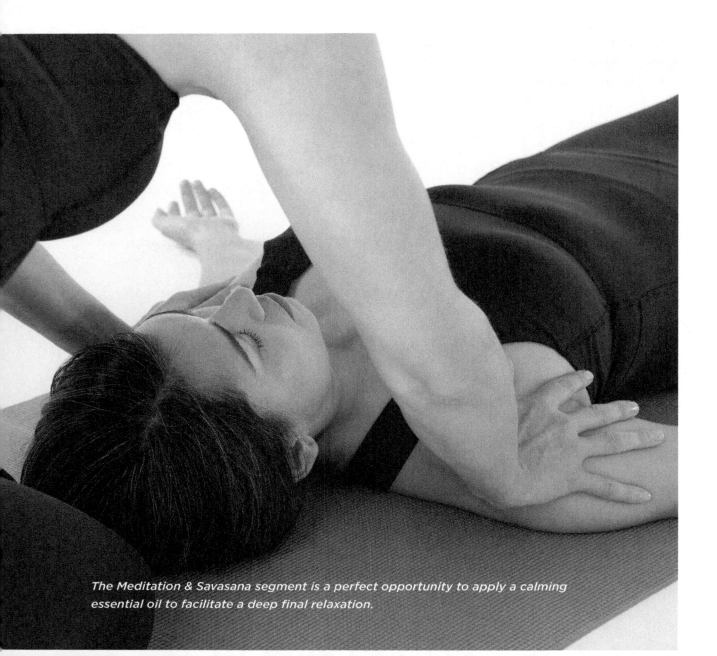

The Meditation & Savasana segment is a perfect opportunity to apply a calming essential oil to facilitate a deep final relaxation.

Workshop Preparation and Sample Script

BASED ON MARCH CURRICULUM

Set-Up Time – Arrive 30-45 Minutes Prior to Workshop

• Prior to your workshop day, enlist assistants to help with oil application during the workshop and staff your dōTERRA information table afterward.

• To make the most of your EssentialYoga workshop, be prepared with the information your students will need to choose their own dōTERRA essential oils, to learn more and to prepare for the next workshop. Stock a dōTERRA information table with the following tools:

  – Invitations and fliers for next events
  – dōTERRA essential oil samples (optional)
  – Reference guidebooks and pamphlets
  – dōTERRA wholesale enrollment forms
  – dōTERRA enrollment kit information
  – Wholesale/Wellness Advocate price sheets
  – Business cards of key contacts
  – Lists of oils used in workshop
  – Paper cups (for students who don't have glass or metal water bottles)

• See "Suggested Room Layout" on page 28.

Check-In

• Start diffuser in practice space.

• Have EVERYONE sign in, even regulars or current dōTERRA users.

    • Offer paper cups to those who don't have glass or metal water bottle.

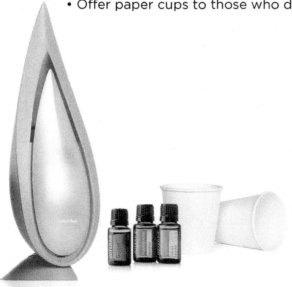

Welcome & Introduction to dōTERRA

- **Assistants begin distributing 1-2 drops grapefruit oil in water bottles or paper cups.**

  SCRIPT: "Welcome to EssentialYoga. My name is _____ and today we are going to start with a 10-minute overview about the essential oils we are going to use today, and then we will begin our practice. After class, we will be happy to answer any questions you may have about the oils for your health and for your yoga practice.

  "We will start with our first oil by giving everyone 1-2 drops of grapefruit essential oil in your water bottle or paper cup to sip on throughout your practice. Grapefruit supports the kidneys and stimulates the lymphatic system while creating a positive mood. One drop of dōTERRA's CPTG Certified Pure Therapeutic Grade oil is equal to almost 30 grapefruit rinds! This is a wonderful way to begin our practice, literally beginning with a 'clean slate.' When using essential oils in your water, be sure to use glass or stainless steel."

- **What are Essential Oils?**

  SCRIPT: "Essential oils are literally a plant's natural defense from disease, predators and weather. When we use essential oils, we are using the plant's defense system for our benefit. There are two primary ways essential oils are collected: Steam distilled and cold pressed. Most plants are steam distilled, while all of the citrus oils are cold pressed from the rind."

- **What Makes dōTERRA Different?**

  SCRIPT: "dōTERRA means 'Gift of the Earth.' CPTG Certified Pure Therapeutic Grade is dōTERRA's certification process that identifies the rigorous testing every batch of oils receives. dōTERRA tests EVERY batch of oils, every time. The reason we can take certain oils internally is specifically related to how pure these oils are. I do not recommend the internal consumption of any other brand of oils – only dōTERRA."

- **Methods of Use**

  SCRIPT: "There are three ways to experience dōTERRA's essential oils: Aromatically, topically and internally. Aromatically, essential oils can directly affect the respiratory system by opening the airways. Aromatic diffusion of oils affects our mood and emotion, and the aroma can purify the air. Today we are diffusing cypress oil, which is beneficial to the respiratory system and helps move stagnant energy through the body. When used topically, essential oils can be applied directly to a specific area (give an example). Many of dōTERRA's CPTG Certified Pure Therapeutic Grade oils can be taken internally. Again, this is because of dōTERRA's rigorous third-party testing that ensures the highest quality and purity of each bottle. When ingested, essential oils can directly support the digestive system and our immune system. As a reminder, we do NOT put essential oils in our eyes, in our ears or in our nose. Be careful not to touch your eyes in our workshop today when we start sharing the oils for you to apply."

- Your Story

  SCRIPT: "Let me start by telling you why I feel so passionate about using the dōTERRA essential oils we are going to share with you today. (Tell your story here but do not discuss major disease "cure" claims – this is to protect yourself and your yoga practice. Why are you doing this? How are you doing this? What results have you, friends, family noticed?) These are my assistants today _____ ."

Centering & Breathwork

- Instructor/Assistants apply **frankincense** topically to brow and back of neck with students lying on their backs. Use ideas from the Workshop Snapshot to set the tone for your workshop during centering or breathwork.

  *SCRIPT: "The next oil we are going to use is **frankincense**, which we will apply to the brow and back of neck. Physically **frankincense** helps to reduce the appearance of scarring, diminishing wrinkles and acne. Scientists are studying **frankincense** for its use with neurological diseases as it is one of the few natural substances that can pass through the blood-brain barrier to better oxygenate the brain. Emotionally it helps one connect to a higher level of consciousness."*

Main Body of Workshop

- Instructor/Assistants distribute 2-3 drops of **marjoram** to be inhaled from hands and self-applied to their neck, shoulders and ankles in EASY POSE.

  *SCRIPT: "Rub your hands together then cup around your mouth and nose. Take several breaths with your eyes closed. Now apply to your neck, shoulders and ankles. Physically **marjoram** helps ease joint stiffness and muscle tension. Emotionally it is the oil of connection and trust to self and others."*

Seated Poses

- Instructor/Assistants distribute 2-3 drops of **Deep Blue blend** to be topically self-applied by students to their lower back, spine and side body in BOUND ANGLE POSE.

  *SCRIPT: "Physically, the **Deep Blue blend** helps ease back, neck and shoulder discomfort. Emotionally it helps one to understand the things that cause us to hurt."*

Meditation & Savasana

• Instructor/Assistants apply **Balance blend** topically to back of neck and shoulders in SAVASANA.

> SCRIPT: *"We will close with **Balance blend** oil in final Savasana. This blend comprises the grounding oils of **spruce, ho wood, frankincense, blue tansy** and **blue chamomile**. On a physical plane **Balance blend** can help with muscle relief and coordination. Emotionally it is calming and strengthens the connection to the lower body."*

End of Workshop & Follow-Up Time

• Lead students out of SAVASANA and close workshop.

> SCRIPT: *"Thank you for coming. If you have any questions or comments we will be available after the workshop. The oils will be available for those who are interested in purchasing at retail or wholesale pricing from _____ . dōTERRA essential oils are a fantastic addition to your natural health choices AND your yoga practice. We hold regular classes at _____ . Our next workshop about essential oils is (announce any relevant future events)."*

Suggested Room Layout

The diagram below is recommended to insure seamless essential oil application during the workshop. Assistants handle application in their rows. The instructor may handle application of a row if there aren't enough assistants. Again, it is highly recommended to have 1 assistant per 6-to-8 students.

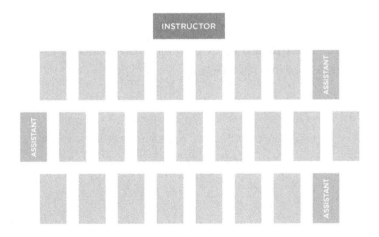

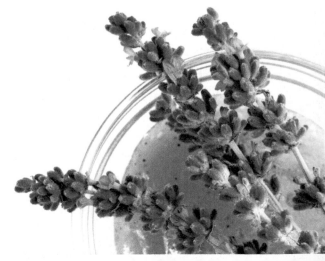

Essential Oil Application In Yoga

Essential oils are applied to various areas of the body depending on the desired result.

There is nothing more nurturing than human touch, and adding this into a yoga practice is one of the reasons many practitioners enjoy attending an EssentialYoga workshop. In The EssentialYoga Program, dōTERRA's CPTG Certified Pure Therapeutic Grade essential oils are applied by the yoga instructor and self-applied by students throughout the workshop as instructed.

When applying CPTG Certified Pure Therapeutic Grade essential oils topically to the student, always convey respect, kindness, sensitivity, confidence/authority and professionalism with a soft, gentle touch of your hands. Be mindful of the laws in your state, province or country as it applies to touching an individual in your workshop. Some jurisdictions require licensing to touch. Note that all oils suggested in the Program can be easily adapted for self-application.

We offer these guidelines to review with students before applying essential oils in your workshop:

- At the beginning of the workshop, always ask permission when applying to a sensitive area (e.g., lower back or neck) and suggest a signal, such as an under-turned corner of the yoga mat, if the student would prefer you not apply an oil in a section of the workshop.

- Be clear and concise about where you will be applying oils, and remind students not to touch their eyes with the oils.

- Let them know you are coming (voice) and in your instruction, explain where you will be applying the essential oil.

- Let them know you are there (hands rubbing together in preparation for application).

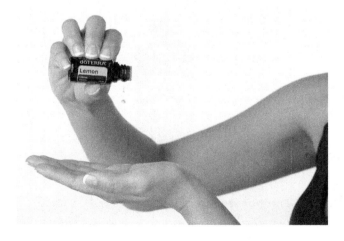

Essential oils are easy to use. Just drip 1-2 drops into your hands and apply topically or rub your hands together and breathe!

Precautions When Applying Essential Oils:

- ALWAYS have **Fractionated Coconut Oil** or some form of vegetable oil handy in your workshop to dilute any oils that cause discomfort to a student. Dilute essential oils with a carrier oil, NOT with water, which spreads the oil.

- When adding essential oils into water, it is best to use a glass or stainless steel container versus plastic or Styrofoam. This is particularly important when using citrus oils, which are able to break down petrochemicals, making them an effective internal detoxifier.

- **Fractionated Coconut Oil** may be combined with the essential oils for ease of application to areas such as the stomach, chest, neck or shoulders.

- Remember to always dilute "hot" oils such as **ginger** and the **On Guard® blend**.

- Use a carrier oil with the **Deep Blue® blend, peppermint, wintergreen** and possibly **AromaTouch® blend** for a smooth and gliding application. Diluting these oils will help temper their potent sensation on the body as they can feel hot to the skin if pores are open in a warm/heated body.

- Pregnant women should not use **clary sage** or blends that contain it.

- Nursing mothers may want to avoid **peppermint** essential oil or blends that contain it.

DEIDRA'S TIP

Essential oils applied by the instructor to the brow, neck, shoulders, spine and low back may be diluted with a carrier oil like dōTERRA **Fractionated Coconut Oil** for ease of application.

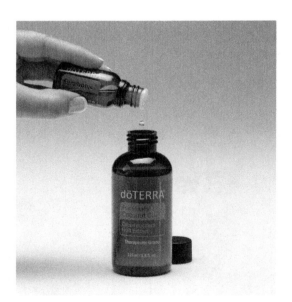

Fractionated Coconut Oil is a great choice because it has no aroma and doesn't stain fabric or yoga mats.

Year-At-A-Glance
EssentialYoga Overview

Use this overview to plan ahead by purchasing the dōTERRA essential oils you will need a month in advance. See Oil Categories and Substitutions for EssentialYoga on page 100 if you do not have the suggested oils.

JANUARY: Vision
Is Your Yoga Practice Aligned with Your Goals?

YOGA FOCUS: Active Flow with twists and inversions

RECOMMENDED OILS: juniper berry, lemon, Roman chamomile, peppermint, InTune™ blend, lavender

ADDITIONAL THEME OPTIONS: Clear Space, Clear Intention/Resolve & Renew

FEBRUARY: Connection
Cultivate an Open Heart

YOGA FOCUS: Active Hatha Yoga with heart openers

RECOMMENDED OILS: ylang ylang, wild orange, frankincense, AromaTouch blend, geranium, Balance blend

ADDITIONAL THEME OPTIONS: Heart Wide Open/Couple's Retreat

MARCH: Alignment
Balance Body, Mind and Spirit

YOGA FOCUS: Head-to-Toe Yin or Restorative

RECOMMENDED OILS: cypress, grapefruit, frankincense, marjoram, Deep Blue blend, Balance blend

ADDITIONAL THEME OPTIONS: Return to Wholeness/Release, Relax, Restore

APRIL: Energy
Capture the Rejuvenation of Spring

YOGA FOCUS: Hatha yoga with twists and forward bends

RECOMMENDED OILS: peppermint, wild orange, lime, cedarwood, rosemary, geranium

ADDITIONAL THEME OPTIONS: Spring Detox/Cleanse Mind, Body, Spirit

MAY: Renew
Receive to Replenish

YOGA FOCUS: Detoxifying Restorative or Yin for kidney/liver meridians

RECOMMENDED OILS: basil, grapefruit, rosemary, myrrh, Zendocrine® blend, frankincense

ADDITIONAL THEME OPTIONS: Seeds of Change/Bloom from Within

JUNE: Breathe
Open to Life

YOGA FOCUS: Vinyasa Flow with focus on side body opening

RECOMMENDED OILS: Elevation blend, grapefruit, lemon, bergamot, juniper berry, lavender

ADDITIONAL THEME OPTIONS: Inhale Citrus, Exhale Calm/Surf the Citrus Wave

JULY: Freedom
Celebrate One's Own Power

YOGA FOCUS: Hatha Yoga with chest and hip openers

RECOMMENDED OILS: eucalyptus, peppermint, frankincense, PastTense® blend, wild orange, Roman chamomile

ADDITIONAL THEME OPTIONS: Sun & Moon/Open & Light

AUGUST: Balance
Creating Optimal Health

YOGA FOCUS: Vinyasa Flow

RECOMMENDED OILS: AromaTouch kit oils (Balance blend, lavender, melaleuca, On Guard blend, AromaTouch blend, Deep Blue blend, wild orange, peppermint)

ADDITIONAL THEME OPTIONS: Tune In & Tune Up/Effort & Surrender

SEPTEMBER: Foundation
Journey Through the Lower Chakras

YOGA FOCUS : Foundation; lower chakra work

RECOMMENDED OILS: clove, cassia, Balance blend, peppermint, cypress, vetiver

ADDITIONAL THEME OPTIONS: Root Down & Be Present/Autumn Equinox

OCTOBER: Release
Surrender and Receive

YOGA FOCUS: Gentle Vinyasa Flow with heart and hip openers, deep forward folds

RECOMMENDED OILS: frankincense, wild orange, Citrus Bliss blend, Elevation blend,
   Serenity blend, Balance blend

ADDITIONAL THEME OPTIONS: Mind, Body, Spirit Connection/Emotional Healing/
   Healing from the Inside Out

NOVEMBER: Gratitude
See the Gift in Your Obstacles

YOGA FOCUS: Heart chakra/heart openers

RECOMMENDED OILS: rosemary, lemon, wild orange, Breathe blend, ginger,
   sandalwood

ADDITIONAL THEME OPTIONS: Heart Full of Gratitude/Radical Gratitude

DECEMBER: Compassion
Cultivate Kindness

YOGA FOCUS: Hip openers and forward bends

RECOMMENDED OILS: Holiday Joy blend, peppermint, frankincense, white fir, thyme,
   wild orange

ADDITIONAL THEME OPTIONS: Cultivate Compassion/Compassion in Action

VISION

1 Vision

Is Your Yoga Practice Aligned with Your Goals?

WORKSHOP SNAPSHOT

What is your vision? Does your practice align with that vision? This workshop invites one to practice with curiosity, while seeking more clarity about where they are and where they want to be. Through twists and inversions one must truly be present with their body and breath. Using oils such as **peppermint** will open the airways and uplift the mood, giving one a "breather" from life's challenges. The **InTune blend** will help balance mental forces with the emotional qualities of the heart. This workshop asks one to explore within, if their practice (Sadhana) is in alignment with their vision or belief (Darshana).

YOGA FOCUS

Active Flow with twists and inversions

RECOMMENDED OILS

Includes cost for this month's workshop.

 DIFFUSE:
JUNIPER BERRY
2 or 3 Drops

$0.89 Retail | $0.66 Wholesale

 LEMON
2 or 3 Drops

$0.16 Retail | $0.12 Wholesale

 ROMAN CHAMOMILE
2 or 3 Drops

$1.56 Retail | $1.17 Wholesale

 PEPPERMINT
2 or 3 Drops

$0.33 Retail | $0.24 Wholesale

 INTUNE BLEND
2 or 3 Drops

$0.81 Retail | $0.60 Wholesale

 LAVENDER
2 or 3 Drops

$0.34 Retail | $0.24 Wholesale

TOTAL WORKSHOP COST PER STUDENT*

$3.20 Retail | $2.37 Wholesale

***Aromatically diffused oil costs are not incorporated into total costs shown.**

> *"The life we want is not merely the one we have chosen and made. It is the one we must be choosing and making."*
>
> – WENDELL BERRY

PORTION OF WORKSHOP	TIME (Minutes)	ESSENTIAL OILS		BENEFITS
Check-In & Set-Up		**JUNIPER BERRY** Diffuse 2-3 drops OR spray room with spritz bottle	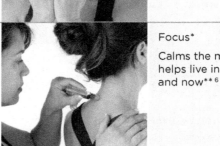	Natural cleansing and detoxifying agent* Helps relieve tension and stress**
Welcome & Introduction To Oils Used In Workshop	10	**LEMON** Add 2-3 drops of oil into glass/metal bottles or paper cup and pass to students	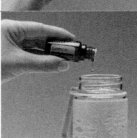	Cleansing and energizing* Increases focus and concentration** 5
Centering & Breathwork	10	**ROMAN CHAMOMILE** Instructor applies to 3rd eye, forehead and back of neck	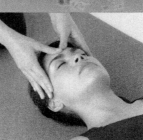	Calms and relaxes* Enhances spiritual awareness**
Main Body of Workshop	40	**PEPPERMINT** Inhale from hands and apply to lower belly OR swipe under tongue before Sun Salutations	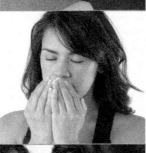	Soothes digestion* Supports assimilation of new information**
Seated Poses	20	**INTUNE BLEND** Instructor applies to forearms while seated before Twist	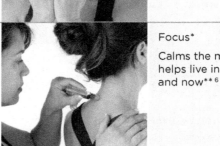	Focus* Calms the mind and helps live in the here and now** 6
Meditation & Savasana	10	**LAVENDER** Instructor applies to 3rd eye, brow swipe and back of neck	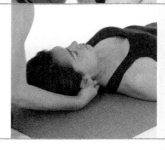	Sedative* Brings one in touch with qualities of open communication and speaking the truth** 7
End of Workshop & Follow-Up				See page 28

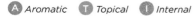 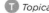

A Aromatic   T Topical   I Internal   *Denotes physical benefits of essential oil. **Denotes emotional benefits of essential oil.

• Seated pose of your choice

• Seated or lying on back

• Sun Salutations
• Lunge with Twist to Wide-Legged Forward Fold to Vinyasa
• Revolved Triangle to Standing Split to Pyramid to Vinyasa
• Handstand or Headstand to Child's Pose
• Down Dog to Standing Forward Fold
• Chair to Twisting Chair

• Sage (Marichi's) Twist
• Seated Forward Fold
• Bridge to Shoulder Stand

• Meditation or final relaxation pose

STEPHANIE'S TIP

As an instructor, if possible, it is helpful to first take an EssentialYoga workshop, and then assist another instructor with oil application before teaching your own workshop. If you don't know of any workshops in your area, you may choose to partner with a friend who teaches or practices yoga, and practice the workshop on each other, or get feedback from the hands-on work with the oils intertwined with the instruction of yoga. It truly is an acquired skill to dance between oil application and teaching the sequence. And just like everything else, you will get better and better each time you do it.

CONNECTION

Connection

Cultivate an Open Heart

WORKSHOP SNAPSHOT

Make the connection with a combination of oils that cultivates an open heart and a quiet mind. Using oils such as **ylang ylang** reconnects one to the pure and simple ways of the heart, while **geranium** helps to foster love and trust. A combination of chest and shoulder openers will leave one feeling energized and more spacious from the inside out. **Frankincense** will connect one to their inner wisdom and encourage trust in oneself and others.

TIP: Consider this for a couples workshop, combining yoga and oils application to deepen the connection to self and to their partner.

YOGA FOCUS

Active Hatha Yoga with heart openers

RECOMMENDED OILS

Includes cost for this month's workshop.

 DIFFUSE:
YLANG YLANG
2 or 3 Drops

| $0.56 Retail | $0.42 Wholesale |

 FRANKINCENSE
2 or 3 Drops

| $1.12 Retail | $0.84 Wholesale |

 AROMATOUCH BLEND
2 or 3 Drops

| $0.42 Retail | $0.30 Wholesale |

GERANIUM
2 or 3 Drops

| $0.44 Retail | $0.33 Wholesale |

 BALANCE BLEND
2 or 3 Drops

| $0.32 Retail | $0.24 Wholesale |

 WILD ORANGE
2 or 3 Drops

| $0.17 Retail | $0.12 Wholesale |

TOTAL WORKSHOP COST PER STUDENT*

| $2.47 Retail | $1.83 Wholesale |

***Aromatically diffused oil costs are not incorporated into total costs shown.**

"When the power of love overcomes the love of power the world will know peace."

– JIMI HENDRIX

PORTION OF WORKSHOP	TIME (Minutes)	ESSENTIAL OILS		BENEFITS
Check-In & Set-Up		**(A)** YLANG YLANG Diffuse 2-3 drops OR spray room with spritz bottle NOTE: Highly aromatic	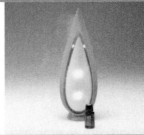	Calms and relaxes* Encourages the heart to experience its full range of emotions** [8]
Welcome & Introduction To Oils Used In Workshop	10	**(I)** WILD ORANGE Add 2-3 drops of oil into glass/metal bottles or paper cup and pass to students	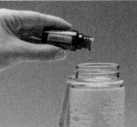	Uplifting* Inspires reconnection to spontaneity, fun and playfulness** [9]
Centering & Breathwork	10	**(T)** FRANKINCENSE Instructor applies to 3rd eye, forehead and back of neck	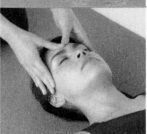	Helps to ground and center the body* Facilitates emotional presence**
Main Body of Workshop	40	**(A)(T)** AROMATOUCH BLEND Inhale from hands and self-apply to back of neck and shoulders before Sun Salutations	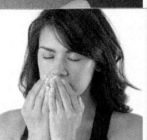	Helps calm anxiety* Moves from stiffness of heart and mind to openness and flexibility** [10]
Seated Poses	20	**(T)** GERANIUM & WILD ORANGE Instructor applies to lower back in Child's Pose *(1 geranium to 3 drops wild orange ratio)*	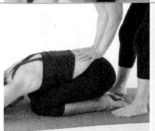	Supports healthy kidney function* Oil of love and trust** [11]
Meditation & Savasana	10	**(T)** BALANCE BLEND Instructor applies to feet		Calming and sedative* Helps to clear the mind and ground the body**
End of Workshop & Follow-Up				See page 28

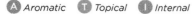 **(A)** *Aromatic* **(T)** *Topical* **(I)** *Internal*   *Denotes physical benefits of essential oil. **Denotes emotional benefits of essential oil.*

• Seated pose of your choice

• Reclined Bound Angle

• Sun Salutations
• Cobra
• Alternating Quad Stretch from Belly to Bow
• Warrior I to Humble Warrior
• Triangle to Pyramid
• Dancer

• Bridge to Upward Facing Bow
• Fish
• Head to Knee
• Happy Baby

• Meditation or final relaxation pose

JANE'S TIP

The yoga mat is a powerful place to bring emotions, truth and awareness to the surface because of the body's connection to the parasympathetic nervous system and the oils' activation of the amygdala, the part of the brain that houses trauma and repressed memories. Yoga and essential oils help to deepen and expedite emotional release, one asana at a time.

ALIGNMENT

③ Alignment

Balance Body, Mind and Spirit

WORKSHOP SNAPSHOT

The selection of oils and the order in which they are used is designed to move stagnant energy, detoxify the body, calm the mind, relax the body and restore equilibrium. A head-to-toe restorative practice of long-held yin poses with a focus on breath, sensation and stillness teaches the power of scent memory. One-to-two-minute hold times starting at the neck, shoulder and wrists then moving to the feet, ankles, thighs and hips begins the process of calming the mind. Moving to the center of the body with passive yin poses held two and five minutes begins the process of relaxing the body. A long, final relaxation combined with **Balance blend** allows the body to assimilate this powerful practice and "align with your core being."

YOGA FOCUS

Yin or Head-to-Toe Restorative

RECOMMENDED OILS

Includes cost for this month's workshop.

 DIFFUSE:
CYPRESS
2 or 3 Drops

$0.25 Retail	$0.18 Wholesale

 GRAPEFRUIT
2 or 3 Drops

$0.26 Retail	$0.18 Wholesale

 FRANKINCENSE
2 or 3 Drops

$1.12 Retail	$0.84 Wholesale

MARJORAM
2 or 3 Drops

$0.31 Retail	$0.24 Wholesale

 DEEP BLUE BLEND
2 or 3 Drops

$1.51 Retail	$1.14 Wholesale

 BALANCE BLEND
2 or 3 Drops

$0.32 Retail	$0.24 Wholesale

TOTAL WORKSHOP COST PER STUDENT*

$3.52 Retail	$2.64 Wholesale

***Aromatically diffused oil costs are not incorporated into total costs shown.**

> "You are not here accidentally – you are here meaningfully. There is a purpose behind you. The whole intends to do something through you."
>
> – OSHO

PORTION OF WORKSHOP	TIME (Minutes)	ESSENTIAL OILS		BENEFITS
Check-In & Set-Up		(A) CYPRESS Diffuse 2-3 drops OR spray room with spritz bottle		Beneficial to the respiratory system* The Oil of Motion and Flow – stagnant energies are brought into motion** 12
Welcome & Introduction To Oils Used In Workshop	10	(I) GRAPEFRUIT Add 2-3 drops of oil into glass/metal bottles or paper cup and pass to students		Assists in clearing kidneys, lymphatic system, vascular system* Enhances a joyful, positive mood**
Centering & Breathwork	10	(A) (T) FRANKINCENSE Instructor applies to 3rd eye, forehead and back of neck		Calms the nervous system* Assists those feeling vulnerable to feel protected** 13
Main Body of Workshop	40	(A) (T) MARJORAM Inhale from hands and apply to neck, shoulders and ankles in seated pose		Helps relieve discomfort of joint stiffness and muscle tension* Oil of Connection and Trust to self and others** 14
Seated Poses	20	(A) (T) DEEP BLUE BLEND Inhale from hands and apply to lower back, spine and side body in Bound Angle		Soothes back, neck and shoulder* The Oil of Surrendering** 6
Meditation & Savasana	10	(T) BALANCE BLEND Instructor cups hand over student's nose and applies to 3rd eye, back of neck and shoulders		Aids in harmonizing body systems, grounding* Calming; strengthens a connection to the lower body**
End of Workshop & Follow-Up				See page 28

See page 28

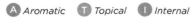

(A) *Aromatic*　(T) *Topical*　(I) *Internal*　　*Denotes physical benefits of essential oil.　**Denotes emotional benefits of essential oil.*

Teach your students the power of scent memory by asking them to cup and hold their hands over mouth and nose with eyes closed. As they take deep breaths through their nose say "Lock this scent in your memory. Use it to remind yourself to come back to your breath, stillness and sensation."

• Seated pose of your choice

• Lying on back

• Comfortable seated pose with movement to open neck, shoulders and wrists
• Cat and Cow
• Standing Forward Fold to Table Top
• Ankle Stretch to Toe Squat
• Reclined Hero
• Down Dog

• Bound Angle Forward Fold
• Banana
• Reclined Spinal Twist

• Meditation or final relaxation pose

ENERGY

④ Energy

Capture the Rejuvenation of Spring

WORKSHOP SNAPSHOT

This workshop was created mindfully to cleanse the mind, body and spirit and make room for the new. **Lime** oil was chosen for its ability to cleanse the heart of emotional toxins combined with a smart sequence of twists and forward bends humbly guiding the body to move out what no longer is needed. **Geranium** is a gentle oil chosen to assist the mind, body and spirit to trust in the process, softening anger and assisting in healing. This detoxifying workshop creates a deep, physical spring cleaning, leaving students feeling rejuvenated from the inside out.

YOGA FOCUS

Hatha Yoga twists and forward bends

RECOMMENDED OILS

Includes cost for this month's workshop.

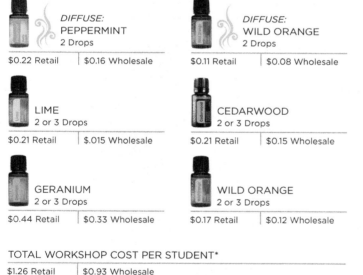
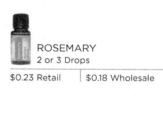

DIFFUSE:
PEPPERMINT
2 Drops

$0.22 Retail | $0.16 Wholesale

DIFFUSE:
WILD ORANGE
2 Drops

$0.11 Retail | $0.08 Wholesale

LIME
2 or 3 Drops

$0.21 Retail | $.015 Wholesale

CEDARWOOD
2 or 3 Drops

$0.21 Retail | $0.15 Wholesale

ROSEMARY
2 or 3 Drops

$0.23 Retail | $0.18 Wholesale

GERANIUM
2 or 3 Drops

$0.44 Retail | $0.33 Wholesale

WILD ORANGE
2 or 3 Drops

$0.17 Retail | $0.12 Wholesale

TOTAL WORKSHOP COST PER STUDENT*

$1.26 Retail | $0.93 Wholesale

***Aromatically diffused oil costs are not incorporated into total costs shown.**

"Just as the caterpillar thought the world was over, it became a butterfly."

– UNKNOWN

PORTION OF WORKSHOP	TIME (Minutes)	ESSENTIAL OILS		BENEFITS
Check-In & Set-Up		**(A)** PEPPERMINT & WILD ORANGE Diffuse 2 drops of each OR spray room with spritz bottle	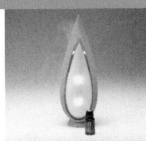	**Peppermint** is a vasodilator and helps to open the airways* **Wild orange** encourages joy and upliftedness** 16
Welcome & Introduction To Oils Used In Workshop	10	**(I)** LIME Add 2-3 drops of oil into glass/metal bottles or paper cup and pass to students	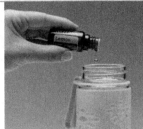	Supports digestion and immunity* Brings balance between the heart and mind** 17
Centering & Breathwork	10	**(A)(T)** CEDARWOOD Inhale from hands and apply to 3rd eye before Child's Pose	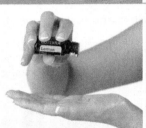	Promotes circulation and helps the body remove toxins* Encourages grounding and focus** 18
Main Body of Workshop	40	**(A)(T)** ROSEMARY Inhale from hands and apply to kidney/liver area in Mountain Pose	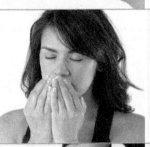	Stimulates memory recall* Aids in times of transition, brings expansion to the mind** 19
Seated Poses	20	**(T)** GERANIUM Instructor applies to arches of feet in Child's Pose	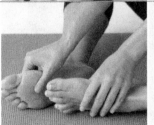	Energizing* Known as the emotional healer** 20
Meditation & Savasana	10	**(T)** WILD ORANGE Instructor applies to 3rd eye, brow swipe and back of neck	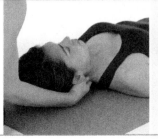	Supports digestion* Calming and uplifting to the mind and body** 21
End of Workshop & Follow-Up				See page 28

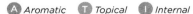

(A) *Aromatic*   **(T)** *Topical*   **(I)** *Internal*   *Denotes physical benefits of essential oil. **Denotes emotional benefits of essential oil.*

One of our hot yoga studio's favorite ways to share the oils on a daily basis is to lightly spritz our students in final savasana with an essential oil.

• Lying on back

• Child's Pose

• Mountain with Standing Side Stretches to Lifted Knee (optional Twist)
• Forward Fold to Pyramid to Revolved Triangle to Standing Splits
• Chair to Eagle to Warrior III to Warrior
• Down Dog to Pigeon add Twist
• Low Lunge to Half Split to Full Split to Forward Fold

• Child's Pose to Thread the Needle
• Revolved Head to Knee
• Reclined Hamstring Stretch to Twist to Long Full Body Stretch

• Meditation or final relaxation pose

RENEW

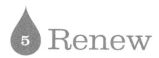

Renew

Receive to Replenish

WORKSHOP SNAPSHOT

This month's oils encourage the release of toxins in the body and mind. **Basil** helps to keep an open mind while **rosemary** helps dispel negativity. The hips are an area we tend to store stress and hold tension. A restorative yin sequence focused on opening the hips stimulates the kidney and liver meridians to clear energetic and physical blockages. Students have the opportunity to experience the power of aromatherapy as a way to stay with intentional breath and focus, to facilitate releasing and softening into their practice. **Myrrh** and **Zendocrine blend** combined with these hip-opening poses encourage the body to "replenish" itself.

YOGA FOCUS

Detoxifying Restorative or Yin for kidney/liver meridians

RECOMMENDED OILS

Includes cost for this month's workshop.

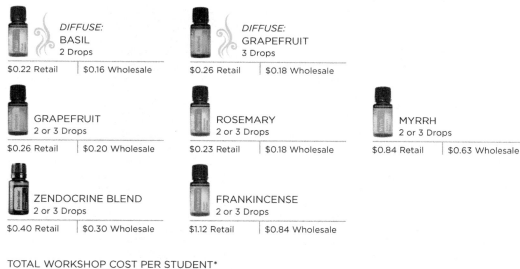

DIFFUSE: BASIL 2 Drops		*DIFFUSE:* GRAPEFRUIT 3 Drops	
$0.22 Retail	$0.16 Wholesale	$0.26 Retail	$0.18 Wholesale

GRAPEFRUIT 2 or 3 Drops		ROSEMARY 2 or 3 Drops		MYRRH 2 or 3 Drops	
$0.26 Retail	$0.20 Wholesale	$0.23 Retail	$0.18 Wholesale	$0.84 Retail	$0.63 Wholesale

ZENDOCRINE BLEND 2 or 3 Drops		FRANKINCENSE 2 or 3 Drops	
$0.40 Retail	$0.30 Wholesale	$1.12 Retail	$0.84 Wholesale

TOTAL WORKSHOP COST PER STUDENT*

$2.65 Retail	$2.15 Wholesale

***Aromatically diffused oil costs are not incorporated into total costs shown.**

> *"In order to carry a positive action we must develop here a positive vision."*
>
> – DALAI LAMA

PORTION OF WORKSHOP	TIME (Minutes)	ESSENTIAL OILS		BENEFITS
Check-In & Set-Up		**BASIL & GRAPEFRUIT** (A) Diffuse 2-3 drops of each OR spray room with spritz bottle	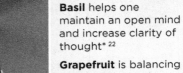	**Basil** helps one maintain an open mind and increase clarity of thought* 22 **Grapefruit** is balancing and uplifting to the mind** 23
Welcome & Introduction To Oils Used In Workshop	10	**GRAPEFRUIT** (I) Add 2-3 drops of oil into glass/metal bottles or paper cup and pass to students	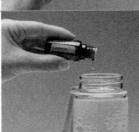	Assists in detoxifying kidneys and lymphatic system* Helps counteract mental exhaustion and frustration** 24
Centering & Breathwork	10	**ROSEMARY** (A)(T) Inhale from hands and apply to chest	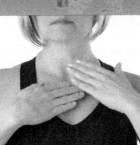	Assists in respiratory health. Helps stimulate the immune system* Encourages positivity** 25
Main Body of Workshop	40	**MYRRH** (A)(T) Inhale from hands and apply to liver before folding forward in Bound Angle	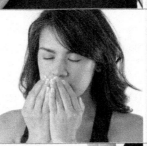	Helps cleanse the liver* Fosters inner stillness and encourages spiritual growth** 26
Seated Poses	20	**ZENDOCRINE** (T) Instructor places 1 drop on each foot arch in Child's Pose and rubs across arches or reflex points associated with kidney	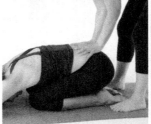	Contains oils for healthy organ support* Encourages letting go of the non-essentials or anything that sabotages** 27
Meditation & Savasana	10	**FRANKINCENSE** (T) Instructor applies to 3rd eye, brow swipe and back of neck	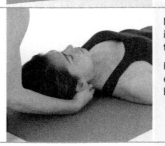	May help decrease inflammation in the body* Helps counteract emotional blockages** 28
End of Workshop & Follow-Up				See page 28

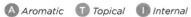 (A) *Aromatic* (T) *Topical* (I) *Internal*   *Denotes physical benefits of essential oil. **Denotes emotional benefits of essential oil.*

• Seated pose of your choice

• Seated cross-legged

• Bound Angle Forward Fold to Windshield Wiper
  Feet and Legs
• Alternating Head to Knee to Wide Angle Seated Forward Bend
• Table Top to Cat and Cow
• Low Lunge to Crescent Moon Lunge
• Down Dog to Child's Pose
• Pigeon to Fire Log to Down Dog to Child's Pose

• Sphinx or Upward Dog
• Reclined Spinal Twist
• Long Full Body Stretch

• Meditation or final relaxation pose

MARTY'S TIP

When preparing for your workshop, you'll want to have enough bottles of each oil on hand for the proper application on the number of students expected. We suggest keeping your "empties" and dripping a full bottle into a few of the empties of that oil or blend. This will allow both the instructor and their assistants to each have a complete set of the oils at the ready to be used during the workshop. If you don't have any empty bottles, consider purchasing some 5ml amber bottles from one of the resources listed in the Appendix to have on hand for just this purpose.

BREATHE

Breathe

Open to Life

WORKSHOP SNAPSHOT

"Let go and open to life" was inspired by dōTERRA's variety of fresh, summer citrus essential oils and their scents. The crisp and uplifting citrus aromas combined with the circular energy movement of this practice are the perfect fit for a seasonal summer vinyasa flow. This workshop focuses on side-body lengthening and healthy function of the kidneys. Combined with the uplifting qualities of citrus oils, this practice creates a powerful antidote to our linear world, helps to remove blinders and opens peripheral vision. Breathe in citrus, exhale into the panoramic view of the body!

YOGA FOCUS

Vinyasa Flow with focus on side body opening

RECOMMENDED OILS

Includes cost for this month's workshop.

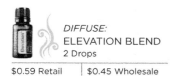

DIFFUSE:
ELEVATION BLEND
2 Drops

$0.59 Retail | $0.45 Wholesale

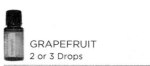 GRAPEFRUIT
2 or 3 Drops

$0.26 Retail | $0.18 Wholesale

LEMON
2 or 3 Drops

$0.16 Retail | $0.12 Wholesale

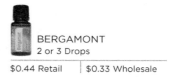 BERGAMONT
2 or 3 Drops

$0.44 Retail | $0.33 Wholesale

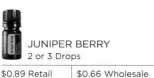 JUNIPER BERRY
2 or 3 Drops

$0.89 Retail | $0.66 Wholesale

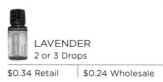 LAVENDER
2 or 3 Drops

$0.34 Retail | $0.24 Wholesale

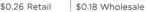
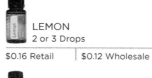

TOTAL WORKSHOP COST PER STUDENT*

$2.09 Retail | $1.53 Wholesale

*Aromatically diffused oil costs are not incorporated into total costs shown.

"How we spend our days is of course how we spend our lives."

– ANNE DILLARD

PORTION OF WORKSHOP	TIME (Minutes)	ESSENTIAL OILS		BENEFITS
Check-In & Set-Up		**ELEVATION BLEND** Diffuse 2-3 drops OR spray room with spritz bottle (A)	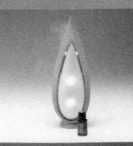	Helps stimulate the body's chemistry when feeling lethargy or sadness* Promotes feelings of self-worth** 29
Welcome & Introduction To Oils Used In Workshop	10	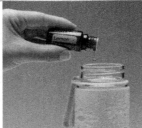 **GRAPEFRUIT** Add 2-3 drops of oil into glass/metal bottles or paper cup and pass to students (I)		Assists in detoxification of the body; helps cleanse the kidneys* Grapefruit teaches true respect and appreciation for one's body** 30
Centering & Breathwork	10	**LEMON** Instructor applies to 3rd eye, forehead and back of neck during reclined poses (T)	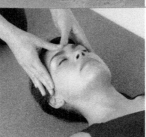	May help increase oxygenation around the pineal and pituitary gland* Oil of focus – this crisp scent improves ability to focus** 31
Main Body of Workshop	40	**BERGAMOT** Inhale from hands and apply to heart area before Seated Pelvic Rotation (A) (T)	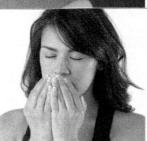	Helps to calm and uplift, energize* Encourages balance, strength and confidence** 32
Seated Poses	20	**JUNIPER BERRY** Inhale from hands and apply to the low back over the kidneys before Child's Pose (A) (T)	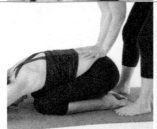	Supports detoxification of the kidneys and may assist with healthy circulation* Elevates one's spiritual awareness** 33
Meditation & Savasana	10	**LAVENDER** Instructor applies as scalp massage (T)	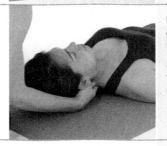	Calming to the psyche and tissue; assists with relaxation* Allows one to share their true self with others** 34
End of Workshop & Follow-Up				See page 28

  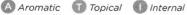 (A) *Aromatic* (T) *Topical* (I) *Internal*   *Denotes physical benefits of essential oil. **Denotes emotional benefits of essential oil.*

I have found that when teaching an EssentialYoga Workshop, students love a longer savasana with lots of hands-on application of the oils. It is a beautiful experience that yogis don't want to see end. Some have said "It feels like spa-yoga".

• Seated pose of your choice

• Reclined Alternating Knee to Chest Pose
* Reclined Hamstring Stretch

• Seated Pelvic Rotation
• Spinal Balance to Table to Star Gazer
• Sun Salutations
• Warrior II to Reverse Warrior to Extended Side Angle to Vinyasa
• Side Plank to Wild Thing to Down Dog to Child's Pose
• Standing Forward Fold to Tree

• Camel
• Revolved Head to Knee
• Bound Angle Forward Fold

• Meditation or final relaxation pose

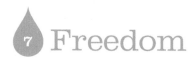 Freedom

Celebrate One's Own Power

WORKSHOP SNAPSHOT

Celebrating one's own innate freedom (Sva Tantria) invites us to remember that no one or no thing can disturb the freedom on the inside unless it is allowed. The practice of hip opening and backbends will create more spaciousness in the body to cultivate this remembrance. These postures, coupled with oils such as **peppermint** to lift the mood and energetically open the heart and **wild orange,** are used to remind us that life should be creative and playful.

YOGA FOCUS

Hatha Yoga with chest and hip openers class

RECOMMENDED OILS

Includes cost for this month's workshop.

 DIFFUSE:
EUCALYPTUS
2 or 3 Drops

| $0.23 Retail | $0.17 Wholesale |

 PEPPERMINT
2 or 3 Drops

| $0.33 Retail | $0.24 Wholesale |

 FRANKINCENSE
2 or 3 Drops

| $1.12 Retail | $0.84 Wholesale |

PASTTENSE BLEND
2 or 3 Drops

| $0.43 Retail | $0.33 Wholesale |

 WILD ORANGE
2 or 3 Drops

| $0.17 Retail | $0.12 Wholesale |

 ROMAN CHAMOMILE
2 or 3 Drops

| $1.56 Retail | $1.17 Wholesale |

TOTAL WORKSHOP COST PER STUDENT*

| $3.61 Retail | $2.70 Wholesale |

***Aromatically diffused oil costs are not incorporated into total costs shown.**

"And the day came when the risk to remain a tight bud was more painful than the risk it took to blossom."

– ANAIS NIN

PORTION OF WORKSHOP	TIME (Minutes)	ESSENTIAL OILS		BENEFITS
Check-In & Set-Up		 **EUCALYPTUS** Diffuse 2-3 drops OR spray room with spritz bottle	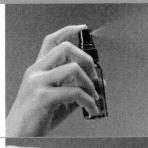	Helps support healthy respiratory function* The Oil of Wellness** 35
Welcome & Introduction To Oils Used In Workshop	10	 **PEPPERMINT** Add 2-3 drops of oil into glass/metal bottles or paper cup and pass to students	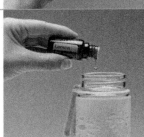	Cooling and supports healthy, normal digestion* Fosters joy, offers reprieve from disappointment** 36
Centering & Breathwork	10	 **FRANKINCENSE** Inhale from hands and apply to chest before Cat and Cow	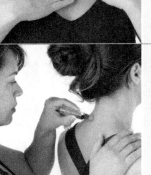	Helps with cell regeneration* 37 Powerful cleanser of spiritual darkness**
Main Body of Workshop	40	 **PASTTENSE BLEND** Instructor applies to base of hairline while lying on belly	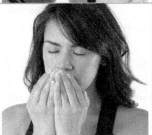	Assists with relief of migraines and headaches* 38 Helps regain equilibrium following periods of fatigue** 39
Seated Poses	20	 **WILD ORANGE** Inhale from hands and apply to belly OR swipe under tongue before Fire Log	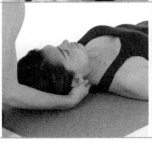	May help with muscle soreness* Encourages self-confidence and positivity** 40
Meditation & Savasana	10	 **ROMAN CHAMOMILE** Instructor applies to 3rd eye, brow swipe and back of neck		May help with muscle tension* Encourages inner peace** 41
End of Workshop & Follow-Up				See page 28

Ⓐ *Aromatic*   Ⓣ *Topical*   Ⓘ *Internal*   *Denotes physical benefits of essential oil.   **Denotes emotional benefits of essential oil.*

• Seated pose of your choice

• Cat and Cow to Child's Pose

• Sphinx to Cobra
• Locust to Down Dog
• Pigeon with Quad Stretch
• High Lunge to Warrior III to Half Moon
• Warrior II to Side Angle to Triangle
• Down Dog

• Bridge or Upward Facing Bow to Alternating Knee
  to Chest
• Fire Log to Cow Face
• Half or Full Lotus
• Happy Baby to Knees to Chest

• Meditation or final relaxation pose

DEIDRA'S TIP

I always have **PastTense blend** roll-on on hand in case I notice students dealing with tight muscle or injuries. It's so easy to walk by and just give them a swipe of oil where needed. They appreciate that additional way to work out tension on the mat!

BALANCE

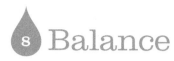

Balance

Creating Optimal Health

WORKSHOP SNAPSHOT

This Vinyasa Flow was sequenced to afford a slower-paced experience of the integration of oils, movement and breath. As the body continues to warm, it will act as its own diffuser, allowing the benefits of each oil to permeate fully. The collection of oils for this workshop were chosen from dōTERRA's **AromaTouch Technique.** To help support the body's system to function optimally, we layer eight essential oils and blends in response to stress, increased toxin levels, inflammation and autonomic nervous system imbalance. Paired with yoga, the oils help the body and mind move toward a holistic state of being.

YOGA FOCUS

Vinyasa Flow

RECOMMENDED OILS

Includes cost for this month's workshop.

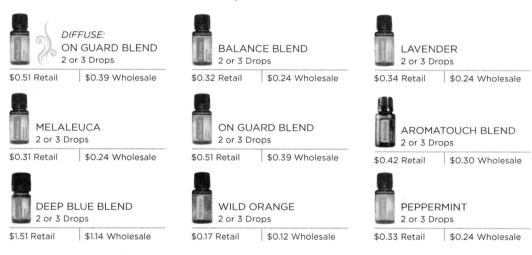

DIFFUSE:
ON GUARD BLEND
2 or 3 Drops

$0.51 Retail | $0.39 Wholesale

BALANCE BLEND
2 or 3 Drops

$0.32 Retail | $0.24 Wholesale

LAVENDER
2 or 3 Drops

$0.34 Retail | $0.24 Wholesale

MELALEUCA
2 or 3 Drops

$0.31 Retail | $0.24 Wholesale

ON GUARD BLEND
2 or 3 Drops

$0.51 Retail | $0.39 Wholesale

AROMATOUCH BLEND
2 or 3 Drops

$0.42 Retail | $0.30 Wholesale

DEEP BLUE BLEND
2 or 3 Drops

$1.51 Retail | $1.14 Wholesale

WILD ORANGE
2 or 3 Drops

$0.17 Retail | $0.12 Wholesale

PEPPERMINT
2 or 3 Drops

$0.33 Retail | $0.24 Wholesale

TOTAL WORKSHOP COST PER STUDENT*

$3.91 Retail | $2.91 Wholesale

***Aromatically diffused oil costs are not incorporated into total costs shown.**

"All healing is first a healing of the heart."

– CARL TOWNSEND

PORTION OF WORKSHOP	TIME (Minutes)	ESSENTIAL OILS		BENEFITS
Check-In & Set-Up		(A)(T)(I) **ON GUARD BLEND** Diffuse 2-3 drops OR spray room with spritz bottle	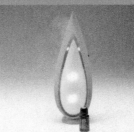	Supports a healthy immune response* Strengthens the inner self** 42
Welcome & Introduction To Oils Used In Workshop	10	(I) **WILD ORANGE PEPPERMINT** Add 2-3 drops of each oil into glass/metal bottles or paper cup and pass to students	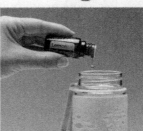	Supports nervous system balance* Uplifting properties that relieve feelings of anxiety and stress** 43
Centering & Breathwork	10	(A)(T) **BALANCE BLEND** Inhale from hands and apply to arches of feet in Bound Angle pose	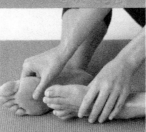	Harmonizes various physiological systems of the body* Promotes tranquility and a sense of balance** 44
Main Body of Workshop	40	(A)(T) **MELALEUCA** Inhale from hands and apply to throat and chest in Mountain pose	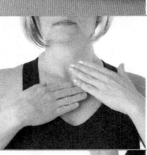	Supports healthy immune response* 45 Oil of Energetic Boundaries – clears negative energetic baggage** 46
Seated Poses	20	(T) **DEEP BLUE BLEND & AROMATOUCH BLEND** Instructor applies to lower back and neck in Child's Pose	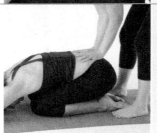	Helps relieve muscle tension and supports decreased inflammation* Calms the mind and helps live in the here and now** 47
Meditation & Savasana	10	(T) **LAVENDER** Instructor applies to 3rd eye, brow swipe and back of neck	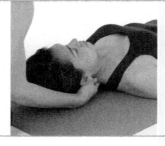	May assist with calming and sedation* Encourages self-care and nurturing self** 48
End of Workshop & Follow-Up				See page 28

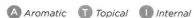

(A) *Aromatic*   (T) *Topical*   (I) *Internal*   *Denotes physical benefits of essential oil. **Denotes emotional benefits of essential oil.

STEPHANIE'S TIP

I find it helpful to teach the same workshop several times at different studios. Then you will really refine the workshops with your own flair and flavor.

- Seated pose of your choice

- Bound Angle Pose
- Cobra to Child's Pose

- Standing Side Stretch
- Sun Salutations
- Low Lunge to Easy Twist to Wide Legged Forward Fold to Horse to Vinyasa
- Warrior II to Reverse Warrior to Reverse Triangle to Vinyasa
- Down Dog to Low Lunge to Lizard
- Hand to Big Toe

- Child's Pose
- Bridge Pose or Upward Facing Bow
- Seated Forward Fold
- Shoulder Stand to Plow to Fish

- Meditation or final relaxation pose

FOUNDATION

⑨ Foundation

Journey Through the Lower Chakras

WORKSHOP SNAPSHOT

"Journey Through the Lower Chakras" helps cultivate a strong physical and emotional foundation. The root chakra is the first chakra and is located at the perineum. It is the root of your being and establishes the deepest connections with your physical body, environment and the earth. This sequence focuses on connecting to the lower chakras with accompanying oils to promote grounding, creativity and inner strength. Meditation and mantra work coupled with the tree oils and roots of **Balance blend** will assist in emotionally connecting with the lower body. Gifts from this month's oils and the poses of the lower root chakras include calmness, patience and a willingness to stay in one place.

YOGA FOCUS

Foundation; lower chakra work

RECOMMENDED OILS

Includes cost for this month's workshop.

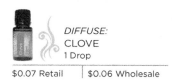

DIFFUSE:
CLOVE
1 Drop

$0.07 Retail | $0.06 Wholesale

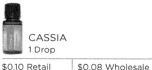

CASSIA
1 Drop

$0.10 Retail | $0.08 Wholesale

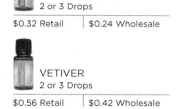

BALANCE BLEND
2 or 3 Drops

$0.32 Retail | $0.24 Wholesale

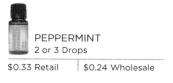

PEPPERMINT
2 or 3 Drops

$0.33 Retail | $0.24 Wholesale

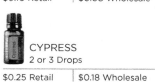

CYPRESS
2 or 3 Drops

$0.25 Retail | $0.18 Wholesale

VETIVER
2 or 3 Drops

$0.56 Retail | $0.42 Wholesale

TOTAL WORKSHOP COST PER STUDENT*

$1.56 Retail | $1.16 Wholesale

***Aromatically diffused oil costs are not incorporated into total costs shown.**

"The deeper the roots, the higher the tree can grow."

– PROVERB

PORTION OF WORKSHOP	TIME (Minutes)	ESSENTIAL OILS		BENEFITS
Check-In & Set-Up		**CLOVE** Diffuse 1 drop OR spray room with spritz bottle		Cleansing* Inspires natural playfulness; clears the head for rational thought**
Welcome & Introduction To Oils Used In Workshop	10	**CASSIA** Add ONLY 1 drop of oil into glass/metal bottles or paper cup and pass to students *(Cassia is a "hot" oil and can irritate those with sensitive lips or mouth – precaution is advised)*		Supports healthy response to pathogenic exposure* Inspires self-assurance in discovering your innate talents** 49
Centering & Breathwork	10	**BALANCE BLEND** Inhale from hands and apply to arches of feet and inner leg		Supports physical balance and calming* A powerful emotional stabilizer, helps to ground energy** 51
Main Body of Workshop	40	**PEPPERMINT** Inhale from hands and apply to lower belly OR swipe under tongue before Low Lunge		May help to open airways; supports healthy digestion* Can offer one a short reprieve from life's difficulties** 52
Seated Poses	20	**CYPRESS** Inhale from hands and apply to heart while seated for twists		Supports lymphatic and circulatory systems* Oil of Motion and Flow, helps to release stagnant energy** 53
Meditation & Savasana	10	**VETIVER** Inhale from hands and apply to arches of feet and inner leg before final relaxation pose		Calming, nurturing* Incredibly supportive in self-awareness work; grounding one in the present moment** 54
End of Workshop & Follow-Up				See page 28

Ⓐ *Aromatic* Ⓣ *Topical* Ⓘ *Internal*   *Denotes physical benefits of essential oil. **Denotes emotional benefits of essential oil.*

SUGGESTED POSES

• Seated pose of your choice

• Low Lunge to Lizard to Down Dog
• Pigeon to Down Dog
• Wide Legged Forward Fold to Frog
• Warrior II to Triangle to Vinyasa
• Squat
• Chair to Boat to Crow

• Core Work
• Sage (Marichi's) Twists
• Reclined Knees to Chest to Twist
• Wide Legged Forward Fold

• Meditation or final relaxation pose

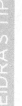

DEIDRA'S TIP

A little sample goes a long way. For an additional $5, give your students the option of walking away with 3 different 10-drop sample vials of oils from your workshop. Have a Modern Essentials book and Emotional Healing with Essential Oils book available so that they can look up other usage ideas for those oils. They get to take part of their EssentialYoga experience home AND learn that one oil can be used for many physical and emotional issues!

RELEASE

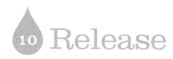 # Release

Surrender and Receive

WORKSHOP SNAPSHOT

One must first release to receive and make space for the new. This workshop helps to increase energy and calm the mind, while the oils assist in emotional healing, releasing stagnant energy, feelings or blockages. Accessible backbend poses are included to assist students in letting go of difficult feelings. Four of the essential oil blends used in this workshop – **Citrus Bliss, Elevation, Serenity** and **Balance** – are part of dōTERRA's Mood Matrix emotional healing oils. This workshop fosters physical, emotional and spiritual healing. The combination of oils and yoga provides a cathartic experience that can be woven into any therapeutic style of yoga to create emotional balance. It is particularly important to hold a safe space for your students in this emotionally opening workshop.

YOGA FOCUS

Gentle Vinyasa Flow with heart and hip openers; deep forward folds

RECOMMENDED OILS

Includes cost for this month's workshop.

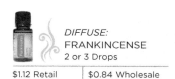 *DIFFUSE:*
FRANKINCENSE
2 or 3 Drops

$1.12 Retail | $0.84 Wholesale

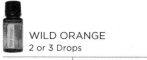 WILD ORANGE
2 or 3 Drops

$0.17 Retail | $0.12 Wholesale

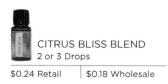 CITRUS BLISS BLEND
2 or 3 Drops

$0.24 Retail | $0.18 Wholesale

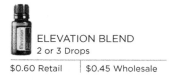 ELEVATION BLEND
2 or 3 Drops

$0.60 Retail | $0.45 Wholesale

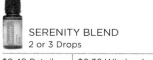 SERENITY BLEND
2 or 3 Drops

$0.48 Retail | $0.36 Wholesale

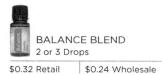 BALANCE BLEND
2 or 3 Drops

$0.32 Retail | $0.24 Wholesale

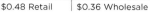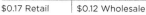

TOTAL WORKSHOP COST PER STUDENT*

$1.81 Retail | $1.35 Wholesale

**Aromatically diffused oil costs are not incorporated into total costs shown.*

"We must embrace pain and use it as fuel for our journey."

– KENJI MIYAZAWA

PORTION OF WORKSHOP	TIME (Minutes)	ESSENTIAL OILS		BENEFITS
Check-In & Set-Up		**FRANKINCENSE** Diffuse 2-3 drops OR spray room with spritz bottle		Supports the body in tissue repair* Brings stability and protection when the heart is feeling vulnerable** [55]
Welcome & Introduction To Oils Used In Workshop	10	**WILD ORANGE** Add 2-3 drops of oil into glass/metal bottles or paper cup and pass to students		Supports healthy digestion; uplifting aroma* Fosters optimism for those who have little tolerance for mishaps or mistakes** [56]
Centering & Breathwork	10	**CITRUS BLISS BLEND** Instructor applies to the back of neck in Child's Pose		Uplifting* Inspires creativity and power by letting go of old limitations and insecurities** [57]
Main Body of Workshop	40	**ELEVATION BLEND** Inhale from hands and apply to the back of neck before Tree Pose		Energizing and stimulating* Assists one in letting go of lower energy vibrations, old habits and addictions; supports self-worth** [58]
Seated Poses	20	**SERENITY BLEND** Instructor applies to neck, shoulders and forearms in Reclined Figure 4		Relaxing, calming* Calms feelings of hostility, fear, anger, jealousy, rage and resentment**
Meditation & Savasana	10	**BALANCE BLEND** Instructor applies to arches of feet		Supports healthy muscle tone* Especially suited for those who seek to escape from life through disconnection or disassociation; grounding**
End of Workshop & Follow-Up				See page 28

See page 28

Ⓐ *Aromatic* Ⓣ *Topical* Ⓘ *Internal*   *Denotes physical benefits of essential oil. **Denotes emotional benefits of essential oil.*

• Seated pose of your choice

• Child's Pose
• Table Top with Lion's Breath

• Mountain with Breath of Joy
• Tree
• Sun Salutation to Cobra to Child's Pose
• Revolved Wide Legged Forward Fold
• Warrior I to Gentle Warrior to Pyramid
• Triangle

• Supported Bridge
• Reclined Figure 4
• Reclined Spinal Twist to Knees to Chest to Legs
  Up the Wall

• Meditation or final relaxation pose

JANE'S TIP

Yoga provides a multi-sensory experience to learn about the oils. When sharing information about essential oils in a yoga workshop, consider sharing both a physical and emotional benefit of each oil to help students become acquainted with the diverse properties of the oils.

GRATITUDE

11 Gratitude

See the Gift in Your Obstacles

WORKSHOP SNAPSHOT

This workshop teaches radical gratitude, allowing one to see the gifts in one's obstacles. Working with backbends and opening the energy of the heart naturally brings one to a place of openness and appreciation. **Lemon** inspires joyful involvement in the present moment, **wild orange** is a reminder of abundance and **sandalwood** inspires individuals to assess where their heart is and challenges them to reorder their priorities to be in alignment with the Universe.

YOGA FOCUS

Heart chakra/heart openers

RECOMMENDED OILS

Includes cost for this month's workshop.

DIFFUSE:
ROSEMARY
2 or 3 Drops

| $0.23 Retail | $0.17 Wholesale |

 LEMON
2 or 3 Drops

| $0.16 Retail | $0.12 Wholesale |

 WILD ORANGE
2 or 3 Drops

| $0.17 Retail | $0.12 Wholesale |

BREATHE BLEND
2 or 3 Drops

| $0.32 Retail | $0.24 Wholesale |

 GINGER
2 or 3 Drops

| $0.47 Retail | $0.36 Wholesale |

SANDALWOOD
2 or 3 Drops

| $2.91 Retail | $2.19 Wholesale |

TOTAL WORKSHOP COST PER STUDENT*

| $3.03 Retail | $4.04 Wholesale |

***Aromatically diffused oil costs are not incorporated into total costs shown.**

> *"If you have only one breath left, use it to say thank you."*
>
> – PAM BROWN

PORTION OF WORKSHOP	TIME (Minutes)	ESSENTIAL OILS		BENEFITS
Check-In & Set-Up		**ROSEMARY** Diffuse 2-3 drops OR spray room with spritz bottle		Supports a healthy immune response; may support better memory and recall* Helps with mental fatigue; lifts spirits and counters depression** 59
Welcome & Introduction To Oils Used In Workshop	10	**LEMON** Add 2-3 drops of oil into glass/metal bottles or paper cup and pass to students		Purifies and energizes the body* Improves ability to focus**
Centering & Breathwork	10	**WILD ORANGE** Inhale from hands and apply to heart area		Supports healthy digestion* Uplifting and stimulating; a great oil for creative thinking** 60
Main Body of Workshop	40	**BREATHE BLEND** Inhale from hands then apply to chest in Mountain Pose		Soothes the tissue of the respiratory system* Deepens the connection to life and invites individuals to let go and receive**
Seated Poses	20	**LEMON & GINGER** Inhale from hands and apply to arches of feet before Bridge		Stimulant; good for digestion and motion sickness* **Ginger** powerfully persuades one to be fully present and participate in life**
Meditation & Savasana	10	**SANDALWOOD** Instructor applies to 3rd eye, brow swipe and back of neck		Stimulates the lymphatic system* 61 Calms, harmonizes and balances the emotions; may help enhance meditation**
End of Workshop & Follow-Up				See page 28

 A Aromatic **T** Topical **I** Internal   *Denotes physical benefits of essential oil. **Denotes emotional benefits of essential oil.

At the end of every EssentialYoga workshop, be sure to not only have paperwork and information ready for anyone who wants it, but also use your workshop as a marketing tool to advertise the NEXT event.

• Seated pose of your choice

• Lying on back with one block under shoulder blades and another under head
• Cat and Cow

• Mountain to Sun Salutations
• Cobra to Locust to Bow
• High Lunge to Low Lunge to Quad Stretch
• Handstand
• Reclined Hero to Down Dog
• Camel

• Bridge or Upward Facing Bow
• Reclined Hand to Foot
• Plow to Happy Baby

• Meditation or final relaxation pose

COMPASSION

12 Compassion

Cultivate Kindness

WORKSHOP SNAPSHOT

Holidays often are a time when our cups become so full that there is little room for anything new. Yoga and essential oils can be a powerful catalyst for emptying our cup to make room to receive. This dynamic hip-opening sequence is combined with seasonal essential oils to make room to receive the many gifts of the season, including self-care and compassion. **Frankincense, white fir** and **thyme** essential oils help cultivate compassion. The uplifting yet calming properties of **wild orange** in final relaxation will remind one of the importance of taking the time to be with oneself in a loving way.

YOGA FOCUS
Hip openers and forward bends

RECOMMENDED OILS
Includes cost for this month's workshop.

 DIFFUSE:
HOLIDAY JOY
BLEND
2 or 3 Drops

$0.39 Retail | $0.30 Wholesale

 PEPPERMINT
2 or 3 Drops

$0.33 Retail | $0.24 Wholesale

 FRANKINCENSE
2 or 3 Drops

$1.12 Retail | $0.84 Wholesale

WHITE FIR
2 or 3 Drops

$0.32 Retail | $0.24 Wholesale

 THYME
2 or 3 Drops

$0.44 Retail | $0.33 Wholesale

  WILD ORANGE
2 or 3 Drops

$0.17 Retail | $0.12 Wholesale

TOTAL WORKSHOP COST PER STUDENT*
$2.38 Retail | $1.77 Wholesale

Aromatically diffused oil costs are not incorporated into total costs shown.

"You have a solemn obligation to take care of yourself, because you never know when the world will need you."

– RABBI HILLEL

PORTION OF WORKSHOP	TIME (Minutes)	ESSENTIAL OILS		BENEFITS
Check-In & Set-Up		**Ⓐ** HOLIDAY JOY BLEND Diffuse 2-3 drops OR spray room with spritz bottle	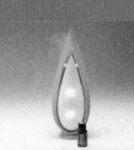	May help reduce airborne pathogens* Helps comfort and soothe emotional well-being**
Welcome & Introduction To Oils Used In Workshop	10	**Ⓘ** PEPPERMINT Add 2-3 drops of oil into glass/metal bottles or paper cup and pass to students	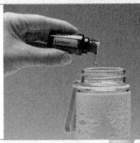	Detoxifying* Uplifting**
Centering & Breathwork	10	**Ⓐ Ⓣ** FRANKINCENSE Instructor applies to arches of feet	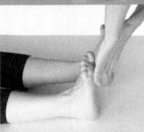	Centering and focus* Helps to create new perspectives based on light and truth** 62
Main Body of Workshop	40	**Ⓐ Ⓣ** WHITE FIR Inhale from hands and apply to chest, throat, back of neck before Tree pose	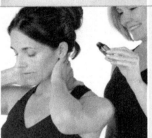	May be beneficial for reducing aches from colds and flu* 63 Creates a feeling of grounding, anchoring and empowerment** 64
Seated Poses	20	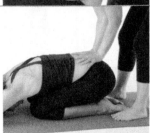 **Ⓣ** THYME Instructor applies to spine in Seated Baby Cradle or Lotus		May help relieve menstrual cramps* The Oil of Releasing and Forgiving; one of the most powerful cleansers of the emotional body** 65
Meditation & Savasana	10	**Ⓣ** WILD ORANGE Instructor applies to 3rd eye, brow swipe and back of neck	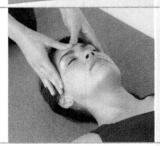	Supports healthy digestion* 66 Supports a positive mood**
End of Workshop & Follow-Up				See page 28

 Ⓐ *Aromatic* **Ⓣ** *Topical* **Ⓘ** *Internal*   *Denotes physical benefits of essential oil. **Denotes emotional benefits of essential oil.*

- Seated pose of your choice

- Child's Pose

- Low Lunge to Diagonal (Down Dog Lunge) to Side Angle to Warrior II
- Tree to Standing Figure 4
- Triangle to Down Dog
- Pigeon to Fire Log to Twist
- Dragonfly Arm Balance
- Down Dog to Child's Pose

- Seated Baby Cradle to Half or Full Lotus with Forward Fold
- Wide Legged Forward Fold
- Reclined Bound Angle

- Meditation or final relaxation pose

JANE'S TIP

EssentialYoga workshops always draw a large crowd at our studio. My dōTERRA team friends and I work closely together to insure a meaningful and unique workshop with the oils each month. Working with others is part of what makes this so fun to offer!

Get Started, Simply!

Sometimes a simple start can help you get more comfortable with the oils in your EssentialYoga Program. Take a look at some ideas on the next page and consider introducing a single oil or blend as you begin your weekly classes. It's an easy way to introduce students to oils throughout the year.

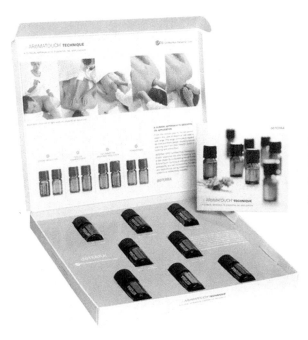

*One suggestion is the dōTERRA **AromaTouch Technique kit.** It is a wonderful collection of eight oils and blends that can be used in many simple ways.*

DEIDRA'S TIP

I've had many opportunities to offer the **Balance blend** to students who have allowed yoga to open them up emotionally on the mat. It's so grounding yet subtle enough to allow them to continue to work through those moments of sitting with difficult thoughts and feelings.

Simple Ways of Introducing Oils Into Your Class

1. Cleanse the Air & Set Mood for Class

Diffuse **wild orange** and **peppermint**, or mix 5 drops of your favorite essential oil with water in a small spray bottle and spritz the room for aromatic benefits.

2. Support Detoxification from the Inside Out

Place 1-2 drops of **wild orange** in stainless steel or glass water bottle and sip.

3. Refine Focus & Centering for Class

Place 1 drop of **Balance blend** on third eye at the beginning of class to bring focus, clarity and spiritual connection to the practice. Applied to the bottoms of the feet, **Balance blend** can bring a sense of grounding and presence to the practice.

4. Activate Energy, Increase Stamina & Open Airways

Diffuse **wild orange** and **peppermint** to create an uplifting and relaxing atmosphere and open the airways.

5. Support Muscles, Joints & Ligaments

Offer **AromaTouch blend** or **Deep Blue blend** topically before, during and after practice.

6. Strengthen Immunity

Apply **melaleuca** to the heart area, front of throat and behind the ears. Instructor-applied **On Guard blend** to the bottoms of the feet as you move toward seated asana.

7. Deepen Meditation & Savasana

Apply **lavender** or **Balance blend** to the temples, brow line, behind the neck and/or feet. Use a combination of **lavender** and **Balance blend** in a spray bottle for a final spritz.

8. Green Clean Your Mats & Studio

Use a combination of **melaleuca** (tea tree oil) in a spray bottle with water to clean and disinfect yoga mats naturally.

9. Dilute & Extend Your Oils

Add a few drops of any essential oil to a carrier oil such as **Fractionated Coconut Oil** and apply by dripping into your hands or with an essential oil roll-on applicator.

10. Personalize Everyday Class/Practice

Choose one oil to work into your class theme or body focus.

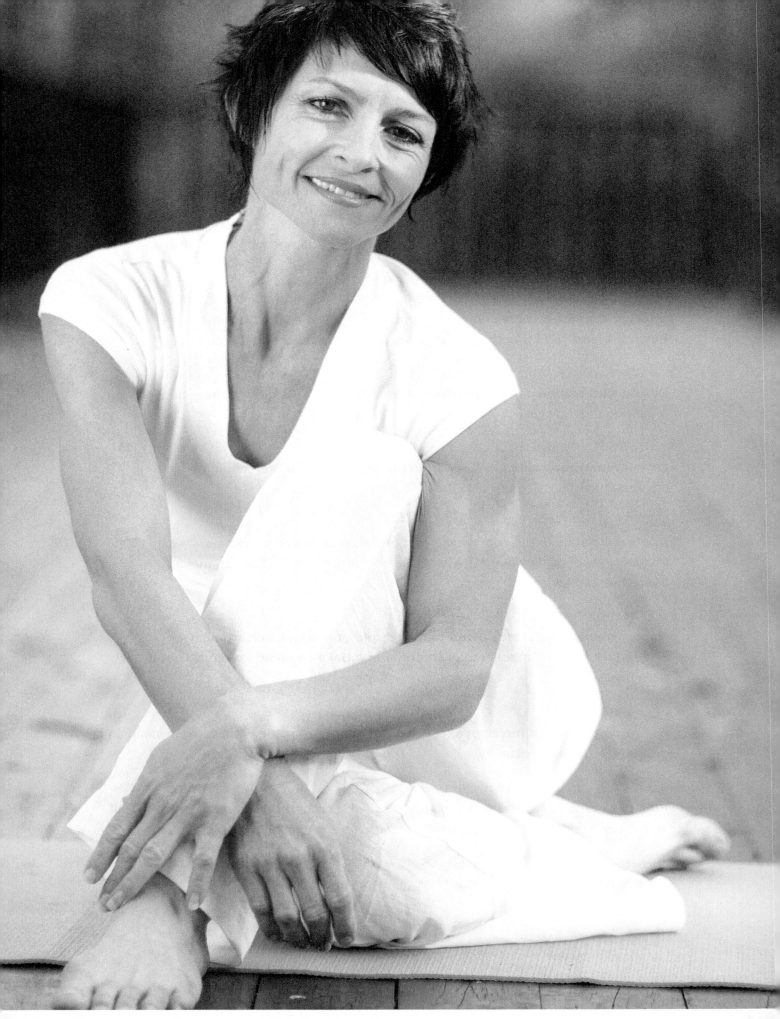

Fuel Your Yoga Passion with Essential Oils from dōTERRA!

There are many ways to supplement your income in support of the yoga practice or business you love, such as taking a part-time job or finding a business partner. But if you have a passion for the essential oils, then join us and dōTERRA to leverage this opportunity to create not only immediate but *lasting* residual income. dōTERRA is a network marketing company – meaning it is designed for each of us to share the oils and products with another person and thereby earn commissions and bonuses for our efforts. As a company, dōTERRA's focus is on educating people about the powerful therapeutic benefits of essential oils and the wonderful complement they make to other natural, healthy lifestyle choices.

Network marketing is a great form of business promotion! Teaching yoga and owning a studio are classic examples of how we market our businesses or classes through networking. We tell people that we teach or own a business and encourage them to come experience it for themselves. We then ask those who support us to bring a friend to class next time. THIS is network marketing at its finest, and it is exactly how dōTERRA oils and wellness products are shared: Person-to-person with one-on-one discussions or in classroom settings, so we can help people learn how to use these beautiful gifts of the earth!

How you earn commissions and bonuses is really quite simple, and can happen literally the week after you become a wholesale member or Wellness Advocate if you share the oils with someone else. Talk to the person who introduced you to dōTERRA and they will be happy to explain how to maximize the Compensation Plan and be paid not only this month, but for literally months and years to come – **creating YOUR "Plan B" of residual, monthly income to fuel your passion and career in yoga.**

To be successful you will need to commit to consistently sharing the oils, teaching others about their benefits, and then showing them how to share and teach. Do this with an open heart. Meet people where they are with natural health tools like essential oils. Do this consistently with a few hours a week and you can build a significant income over a two- to-three-year period. Don't misunderstand – this isn't a magic solution and it isn't always easy. But if you are willing to "show up for work" at building your dōTERRA business with the same commitment you'd give to your own studio or to an employer, and if you are committed to making it work – you WILL be successful! There are many, many of us who have done it ourselves and are happy to help you learn how to create a meaningful, honorable, lasting income for yourself to support your yoga career or studio.

There are three typical pathways people tend to follow toward their goals with dōTERRA. *Which one sounds like you?*

Cover your costs and pay for oils used for personal and in-class or workshop use. We all know that you have to teach a lot of yoga classes to earn a good living. By consistently sharing dōTERRA oils with others on a part-time basis, most people find they can earn enough to offset the cost of their oils and more.

Part-time income to pay for your materials, time and allow you to still teach and practice while saving for a 'Plan B' income. If you're one of the instructors looking for a way to pay big monthly bills – such as your mortgage, car payment, continuing education or outstanding debt – the opportunity is there for you by working 10-20 hours a week for a few years to build a dōTERRA business.

Full-time income to own a studio that you love, plus some time to enjoy your practice along with the financial freedom to choose how and where you live your life. You may not start out at this level of commitment, because it takes a full-time effort to get to this level of earning over a few years. But if you dream of building your own business, owning a beautiful home or traveling the world, this may be the path for you. Many of us are doing this now, and still are able to keep the practice and business we love. In fact, our dōTERRA income helps us keep our studio afloat in leaner months. dōTERRA essential oils are such a perfect complementary business to studio ownership.

> **JANE'S TIP**
>
> When I was first asked if I would like to share dōTERRA oils with others, I was skeptical. I had a brief stint in sales and realized quickly it was not for me. Once I started using dōTERRA oils in my yoga classes, I quickly realized that it was not about "selling" oils but rather "sharing." The oils create an immediate positive impact on people and sharing the oils was a natural part of the work I was doing in helping others find emotional and physical health as a counselor and yoga instructor. Yoga provided a natural environment from which to share with others, and much to my surprise, dōTERRA became a secondary and now primary source of income for my family. Valuing altruistic work, dōTERRA is the perfect fit for my other professions and has allowed me to move in new and exciting directions while sharing these "gifts of the earth".

Instructors:

What's Your "Plan B"?

How dōTERRA Oils Support Your Yoga Livelihood

One typically becomes a yoga instructor because of their passion for sharing what yoga has done in their own lives. Sharing that passion is the next step that leads you to the front of the room. Often the question of "Can I live on what I earn teaching?" doesn't really pop up at that time. In fact, most yoga instructors teach because of their love for yoga, not because they believe it will make them wealthy.

If you haven't asked yourself these honest questions lately, take a minute to do so now:

How can I earn enough money teaching yoga to support this work I love?

What's my "Plan B" if something unexpected happens to my health and I can no longer teach yoga?

Don't let yourself become another yoga instructor statistic…out before your five-year anniversary. Now that you're here teaching and loving what you do, you need to recognize that financing your chosen profession is important so you can continue to teach and share the benefits yoga brings with others.

dōTERRA essential oils offer you a way to earn an honorable income that supports the work you love. dōTERRA essential oils truly complement any yoga practice – on or off the mat.

Think about how you were introduced to the oils. Think about your reactions, what the oils smelled like, felt like, what you may have noticed when they were diffused around you or applied to you. If you enjoyed this experience, then replicate the sharing of the oils to your students and friends in the same way they were offered to you. Have samples handy and share them freely. Remember, this is an experience-based business and people must try the oils to understand their value and to choose them for their own.

Using essential oils is a choice, just like all good, healthy habits – fresh food, clean water, thorough rest, laughter, moving your body and centering your mind and embracing a yoga practice.

Most of us have found that if we approach others with enthusiasm for all good health choices - oils included – many who choose self-care will join our dōTERRA business and follow nature's path to a healthier lifestyle, both on and off the mat.

Then often without even realizing it, we've created our **"Plan B."**

Approaching Studios to Teach EssentialYoga Workshops

Many studio owners are looking for unique workshops to offer their clients. EssentialYoga makes a wonderful addition to any monthly workshop lineup. As outlined in our guidebook, there are 12 themed workshops you can present, along with suggested pricing, staffing and studio timeframes needed. Review this guidebook thoroughly before you approach your next studio owner, and be clear about your workshop intention to:

• Introduce the concept of essential oils and yoga via a monthly theme.

• Use essential oils aromatically, topically and internally for those who wish in the workshop.

• Assist in promoting and marketing the workshop to ensure maximum participation.

• After the workshop, encourage participants to attend a regularly scheduled essential oil class.

• After the workshop, encourage participants to purchase dōTERRA essential oils through you or the studio – depending on your arrangements prior to the workshop (see the person who introduced you to dōTERRA to better understand workshop enrollments and retail sales options).

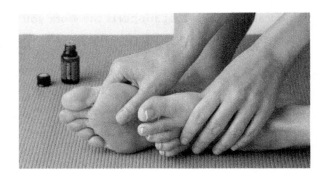

Essential oils applied to the arches of the feet can help students feel emotionally grounded. The oils are drawn into the lymphatic and circulatory systems, creating whole-body therapeutic benefits because the feet have many pores.

Remember that when working with yoga studios, you are not just sharing and promoting the use of dōTERRA essential oils, but also offering a comprehensive service and partnership with the yoga studio that will provide ongoing trainings, workshops and support. Yoga studios that endorse dōTERRA essential oils will carve out a special niche for their studio as one that offers a personal touch and care to all students. **Using dōTERRA essential oils can provide a valuable second stream of income to the studio.** Plus, the training and support to build your dōTERRA business is free and much of it available 24/7 online. What other company helps you build your business with FREE business training?

Owners:

Adding dōTERRA to Your Studio

dōTERRA essential oils and wellness products offer a complementary and profitable addition to the retail product choices you carry at your studio. As CPTG Certified Pure Therapeutic Grade tested essential oils, they are truly the highest quality essential oils in the world (see the section titled *The dōTERRA Difference? CPTG Certified Pure Therapeutic Grade®*). Business owners throughout the country are proud to offer these effective, therapeutic healing tools to their clientele, and have found great success in repeat sales. Why? Because dōTERRA oils work!

A small monthly investment will repay itself multiple fold as you see retail sales increase, clients and instructors staying healthier and enjoying "something different" about your studio as these aromatic healing tools bring a higher energetic vibration. With dōTERRA essential oils, you'll be creating a unique "persona" for your studio – one that is memorable, attractive and a place where others want to spend more time and learn ways to stay well. Using the suggestions in this guidebook, you'll find dōTERRA will help you to:

- Keep clients happy and loyal to your studio

- Offer a unique and healthy setting to practice yoga

- Run a profitable business and secondary income stream that allows you to be paid outside of your teaching income

- Minimize absenteeism of instructors

- Extend your "brand" beyond yoga and into holistic healing with regular essential oil classes

MARTY'S TIP

I carried five other commercially available lines of essential oils for several years in my wellness center. We diffused them, we offered them to clients in our massage treatments and they were available for sale, although few were actually sold. Once I introduced the dōTERRA oils, I was amazed how people were drawn to their significantly cleaner aromas and the immediate therapeutic effect their oils seemed to create. dōTERRA rapidly became my top-selling retail item, and in a time in our economy where everyone was cutting back or going without, their healing properties became the "medicine of choice" for most of my clients. I am forever grateful to the woman who introduced me to them – they literally saved my practice!

How to Incorporate dōTERRA Oils and Wellness Products

Diffuse the Oils at the Reception/Retail Area

dōTERRA offers three diffuser styles that effectively disperse the emotional and physical health benefits of the oils into an area of up to 1,200 square feet. Just a few drops in the diffuser will help keep you, your instructors and clients healthy year-round. The scent memory you will create through continuous, daily diffusing of dōTERRA essential oils will have a profound emotional impact on everyone. Aroma is a powerful tool that can transport us and our emotions to a place of calm and serenity within seconds.

Display Oils for Sampling on the Counter

There are several space-saving and professional wooden and metal display racks available for purchase from vendors listed in the Appendix. Most wellness center owners save empty bottles and use these as counter displays. Clients can sample the scent without an extensive cost to the business owner.

Create a Germ-Free Environment

Provide an opportunity for clients and staff to experience some of the other wellness products and keep everyone healthy! Use the **On Guard Foaming Hand Wash** in your restrooms. Clean surfaces with the **On Guard Concentrated Cleaner.**

Diffuse in the Studio Rooms

Provide a diffuser for instructors in each studio with a simple citrus oil such as **wild orange, grapefruit, lemon** or **bergamot** to cleanse the space and create the scent memory.

Green Cleaning of Yoga Mats

Spritz yoga mats after class by providing a water spray bottle with a few drops of **melaleuca** or **Purify cleansing blend.**

Retail Selection

Depending on your market, you know the price point that most clients will spend for additional items or for class fees. Top sellers often include:

- Introductory Kits (**lavender, lemon** and **peppermint** oils with a CD containing tips on usage)
- **Deep Blue Rub** for muscle aches and strains
- Emotional/mood oil blends of **Balance, Citrus Bliss, Elevation** and **Serenity**
- **On Guard Throat Lozenges, beadlets** and other products
- **PastTense blend** for roll-on easing of migraines, headaches and tense muscles
- **Fractionated Coconut Oil** and unscented body lotion for diluting oils and applying topically

Supporting Products

In addition to the oils themselves, below we have listed a few worthwhile inventory items to carry in your retail area. These tools support the knowledge, use and application of essential oils for your clients. Details on where to purchase are available in our Appendix/Reference section.

- *Modern Essentials* reference books

- *Emotions & Essential Oils – Emotional Reference Guide*

- Diffusers

- Spray bottles

- Booklets about dōTERRA oils

Offer Free Essential Oil Classes

Free weekly classes about dōTERRA essential oils help your clients to learn more about holistic living. Consider addressing a common health concern (sleep, nutrition, sports recovery) or offer an in-depth exploration of a specific oil or blend during your class. Free and low-cost course material is readily available, or be creative and make your own curriculum. Most of us have found that education is the key when using essential oils, and there is always more we can learn together!

Instructor Training Programs

Incorporating an essential oil module into your structured instructor training program is a wonderful idea! Need help? Contact any of the authors of this guidebook for information about your next training session and for options on in-depth weekend essential oil and yoga workshop opportunities for your studio.

Apply essential oils that bring the attention back to intentional breath as an aid to sinking into challenging poses such as Half Pigeon.

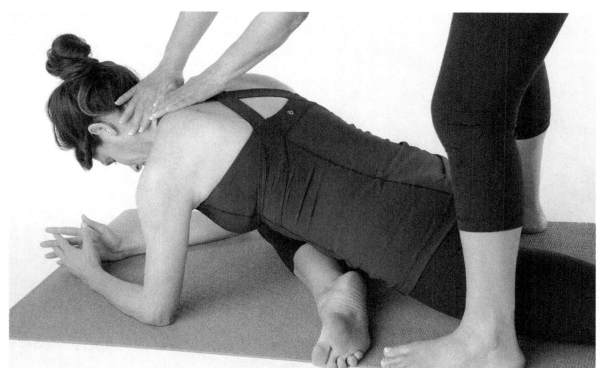

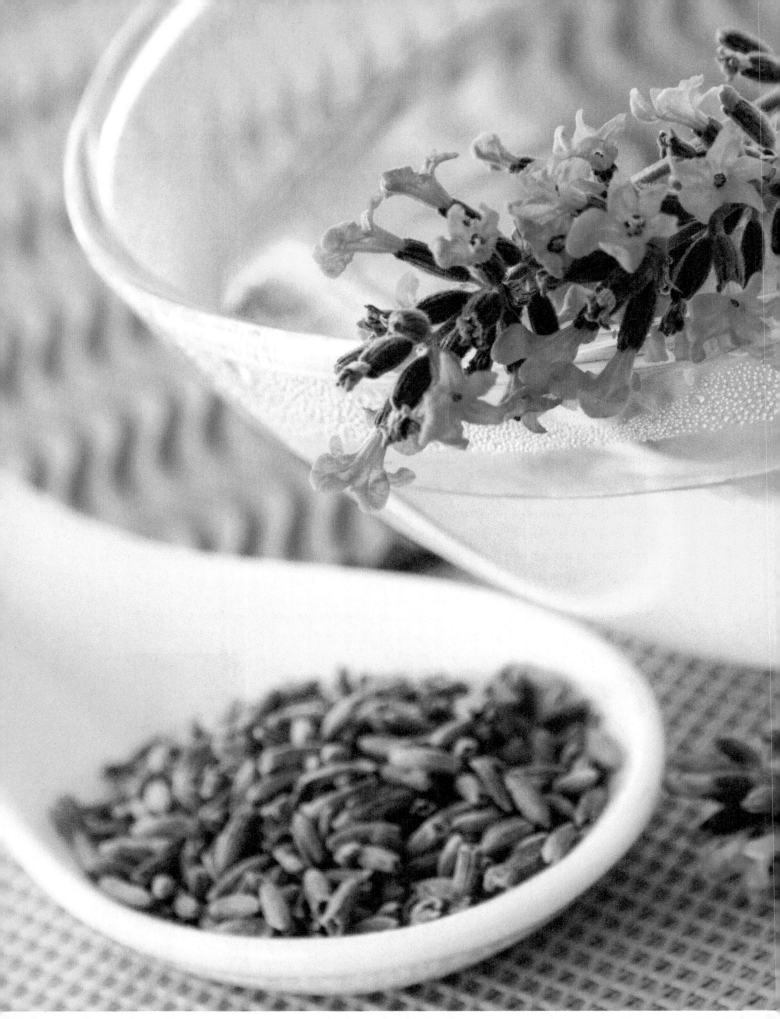

Purchasing Options

dōTERRA truly honors our ability to decide what is best for us and provides several great choices in how we purchase our essential oils and wellness products. Choose the method that fits your needs to get started!

Wholesale Member/Wellness Advocate

- 25% discount off retail

- 2 free websites provided – one wholesale buying site, one retail site for your customers

- Optional Loyalty Rewards Program earns up to 30% in free product credits monthly

- Monthly 10% savings on a featured product

- FREE monthly Product of the Month option

- Opportunity to earn commissions and bonuses if monthly order exceeds 100 PV (point value)

- Choose a pre-determined Enrollment Kit for extra savings, or build your own kit by paying a $35 annual membership fee

- **BEST FOR:** Anyone who wants the best price and/or who is interested in residual income as a supplemental or complementary business opportunity with dōTERRA.

Preferred Member Option

- $10 one-time fee

- 20% discount off retail

- No websites, commissions or bonuses earned

- Allowed as a 2nd account from the same person

- **BEST FOR:** Studio owner who uses their Wellness Advocate/wholesale account for personal purchases and their Preferred Member account for retail purchases as a separate entity; those who want a "deal" but don't want to become wholesale members yet (Preferred Members CAN upgrade their account to become a Wellness Advocate).

Retail Option

- **BEST FOR:** Trialing products.

Your dōTERRA Support Team

You have several sources of support to learn more about the oils and using them in your practice. The person who introduced you to the oils can help you enroll as a wholesale member/Wellness Advocate with dōTERRA. In addition, please note these support resources specifically for you:

When you enroll with dōTERRA or purchase this guidebook, you will have personal support and guidance on how to use essential oils, free on-line and local training classes, on-line resources, workshops on how to implement and teach with essential oils, continuous follow up, and customer service in helping you grow your dōTERRA business with your studio. **What other product can a studio purchase where they are getting free, ongoing consultations to help them grow THEIR business?**

dōTERRA Customer Service department **800-411-8151** is available Monday through Saturday.

dōTERRA's key website is **www.dōTERRAeveryday.com**. Here you'll find training, education, tips on getting started with the business, and a daily blog with product and business tips.

Scientific research can be found at **www.aromaticscience.com**.

Online webinars and training are available through **www.oilsmentor.com** as well as multiple team websites. Ask your Enroller/Sponsor for ideas.

Teach the Teachers: Contact the authors of The EssentialYoga Program or go to our website to learn more about our training workshops for your staff: **www.essentialyogaprogram.com**.

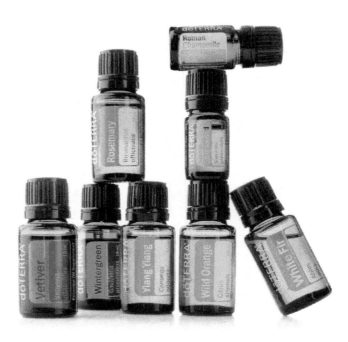

Launching Your EssentialYoga Program

Marketing Your Workshops

Probably *the* most important aspect of a successful EssentialYoga workshop is the promotion or marketing of your upcoming event, followed by your energy and enthusiasm for what students will experience in the workshop.

Most of us who have taught EssentialYoga workshops have found that many NEW students come to them. *So think outside the box!* Use these workshops to expand your reach within your local community and to attract those new to yoga to explore a safe and gentle style of learning that welcomes them into aromatic bliss!

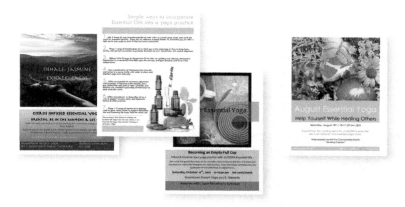

Below is a simple and effective suggested checklist you may want to use and add to your own proven approaches.

Marketing Checklist:

- ☐ Determine workshop cost, maximum number of students, date and time
- ☐ Post a workshop flier in the studio (front desk, front door, restrooms)
- ☐ Offer mini fliers about the workshop to current clients and encourage them to attend!
- ☐ Post it on the studio website workshop calendar, as well as on the studio's social media pages
- ☐ Keep fliers in your purse or bag to share with friends outside the studio
- ☐ Text a reminder to key people who've expressed interest a few days before the workshop
- ☐ Call your key clients and make sure they've signed up to attend!

Take EssentialYoga to Town!

Remember that this type of program is truly unique to offer to groups in your community who may be looking for something really different for their next gathering or event. Think about approaching some non-traditional organizations about offering an EssentialYoga Program workshop specifically designed for:

- Hotel sales staffs about offering a gentle or restorative class option for their meeting groups and/or their spouses
- Chair yoga options for veterans groups or local senior citizen centers
- Middle and high school students for health class, plant biology class or after-school event
- College dance students
- Church or local groups interested in natural health ideas
- Yoga instructor training programs
- Gather neighbors and friends together for a fun summer, outdoor EssentialYoga workshop!

For more marketing ideas, visit our website **www.essentialyogaprogram.com.**

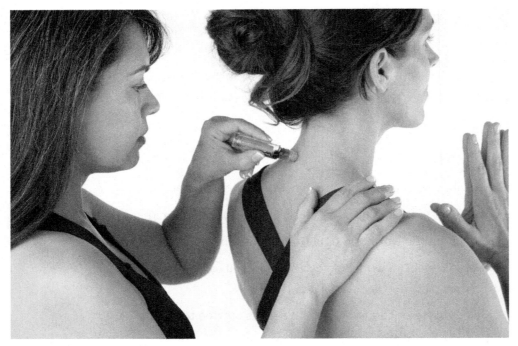

Roll-on essential oil bottles help speed application during a large workshop of students. The antiseptic/antibacterial nature of essential oils makes them very safe for repeated topical application.

dōTERRA Essential Oil Pricing

There are as many philosophies about what to charge for an EssentialYoga workshop as there are forms of yoga! You will need to decide what works best for you, but DO take a few moments as you begin planning your workshop to think about which oils and how you will be using them in your EssentialYoga workshop. Some studios choose to take an average cost of all 12 workshops and add a standard monthly workshop materials fee. You will have your own marketing approach to pricing into which you'll want to include the cost of oils for your workshop.

On the next page is a chart of wholesale prices (best pricing) for your oils. Think about which oils you will be diffusing. Will you pre-dilute the oils you apply topically to your students, or will you give them 1 or 2 drops "neat" in their hand? Once you have identified this information, tally the costs and add a bit for the unexpected. To give you an idea, we have provided estimated costs for each monthly workshop in our guidebook that you'll find on each month's introduction page.

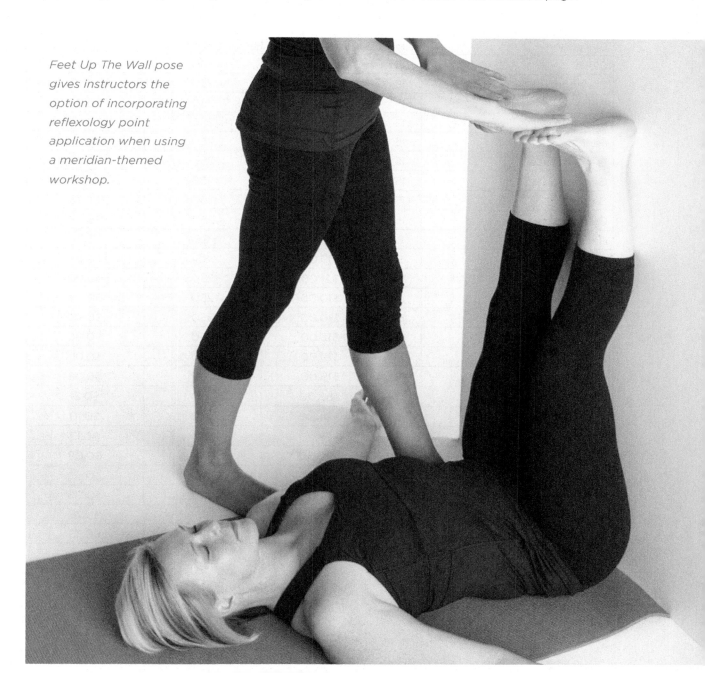

Feet Up The Wall pose gives instructors the option of incorporating reflexology point application when using a meridian-themed workshop.

dōTERRA Wholesale Oil Costs

(Based on pricing effective March 1, 2014 [67])

BASED ON 250 DROPS PER 15 ML BOTTLE
AND 85 DROPS PER 5 ML BOTTLE

OILS				
	ML	COST PER BOTTLE	DROPS PER BOTTLE	COST PER DROP
Basil	15	$20.00	250	$0.08
Bergamot	15	$27.50	250	$0.11
Black pepper	5	$22.00	85	$0.26
Cassia	15	$19.00	250	$0.08
Cedarwood	15	$13.00	250	$0.05
Cilantro	15	$26.00	250	$0.10
Cinnamon	5	$21.00	85	$0.25
Clary sage	15	$36.50	250	$0.15
Clove	15	$14.00	250	$0.06
Coriander	15	$26.00	250	$0.10
Cypress	15	$15.50	250	$0.06
Eucalyptus	15	$14.00	250	$0.06
Fennel	15	$15.00	250	$0.06
Frankincense	15	$69.75	250	$0.28
Geranium	15	$27.00	250	$0.11
Ginger	15	$29.00	250	$0.12
Grapefruit	15	$16.00	250	$0.06
Helichrysum	5	$75.00	85	$0.88
Juniper berry	5	$19.00	85	$0.22
Lavender	15	$21.00	250	$0.08
Lemon	15	$10.00	250	$0.04
Lemongrass	15	$10.00	250	$0.04
Lime	15	$13.00	250	$0.05
Marjoram	15	$19.00	250	$0.08
Melaleuca	15	$19.00	250	$0.08
Myrrh	15	$52.00	250	$0.21
Oregano	15	$24.00	250	$0.10
Patchouli	15	$29.50	250	$0.12
Peppermint	15	$20.50	250	$0.08
Roman chamomile	5	$33.00	85	$0.39
Rosemary	15	$14.00	250	$0.06
Sandalwood (Indian)	5	$61.75	85	$0.73
Sandalwood (Hawaiian)	5	$61.75	85	$0.73

OILS				
	ML	COST PER BOTTLE	DROPS PER BOTTLE	COST PER DROP
Thyme	15	$27.50	250	$0.11
Vetiver	15	$34.50	250	$0.14
White fir	15	$20.00	250	$0.08
Wild orange	15	$10.50	250	$0.04
Wintergreen	15	$16.00	250	$0.06
Ylang ylang	15	$35.25	250	$0.14

BLENDS				
	ML	COST PER BOTTLE	DROPS PER BOTTLE	COST PER DROP
AromaTouch blend	15	$26.00	250	$0.10
Balance blend	15	$20.00	250	$0.08
Breathe blend	15	$20.00	250	$0.08
Citrus Bliss blend	15	$15.00	250	$0.06
Clary Calm blend	10	$24.50	170	$0.14
Deep Blue blend	5	$32.00	85	$0.38
DigestZen® blend	15	$31.00	250	$0.12
Elevation blend	15	$37.00	250	$0.15
Holiday Joy blend (available seasonally)	15	$24.50	250	$0.10
Immortelle blend	10	$69.50	170	$0.41
InTune blend	10	$34.50	170	$0.20
On Guard blend	15	$32.00	250	$0.13
PastTense blend	10	$18.50	170	$0.11
Purify blend	15	$18.00	250	$0.07
Serenity blend	15	$30.00	250	$0.12
Slim & Sassy™ blend	15	$24.50	250	$0.10
TerraShield® blend	15	$9.50	250	$0.04
Whisper blend	5	$24.00	85	$0.28
Zendocrine blend	15	$24.50	250	$0.10

Oil Categories and Substitutions for EssentialYoga

As you review the monthly curriculum, you may choose to substitute an oil with your own preference or you may not have as much of an oil available for your workshop as you thought. Simply check the physical and emotional benefits listed in a particular month's curriculum, then find the single oil or blend from a similar category below to substitute.

GROUNDING	UPLIFTING & BREATHWORK	CALMING	MEDITATIVE & CENTERING	ENERGIZING	DETOXIFYING	PHYSICAL COMFORT	IMMUNE BOOSTING
Balance	AromaTouch	AromaTouch	Balance	Breathe	Cassia	AromaTouch	Basil
Cedarwood	Bergamot	Balance	Cedarwood	Citrus Bliss	Cilantro	Basil	Bergamot
Clary Sage	Breathe	Clary Calm	Clary Calm	Elevation	DigestZen	Black Pepper	Cinnamon
Cypress	Citrus Bliss	Frankincense	Frankincense	Eucalyptus	Fennel	Coriander	Clove
Frankincense	Cypress	InTune	Helichrysum	Grapefruit	Geranium	Deep Blue	Frankincense
Geranium	Elevation	Lavender	Immortelle	Juniper Berry	Ginger	Eucalyptus	Lemon
Juniper Berry	Eucalyptus	Lemon	InTune	PastTense	Grapefruit	Frankincense	Lemongrass
Myrrh	Grapefruit	Patchouli	Lemon	Peppermint	Lemon	Lavender	Melaleuca
Patchouli	Lemon	Roman chamomile	Lemongrass	Rosemary	Lemongrass	Lemongrass	Myrrh
Sandalwood	Lime	Sandalwood	Patchouli	Slim & Sassy	Lime	Marjoram	On Guard
Vetiver	Past Tense	Serenity	Roman chamomile	Thyme	Patchouli	PastTense	Oregano
Ylang Ylang	Peppermint	Vetiver	Sandalwood	White Fir	Purify	White Fir	Thyme
White Fir	Wild Orange	Whisper	Vetiver	Wild Orange	Zendocrine	Wintergreen	Zendocrine

Appendix & References

Sources Referenced in this Guidebook:

Websites:

http://theida.com/ew/wp-content/uploads/2010/10/Aromatherapy-Applications-for-Yoga-Practice.pdf

Reference Books:

Modern Essentials – A Contemporary Guide to the Therapeutic Use of Essential Oils
AromaTools, 2013

Emotions & Essential Oils – A Modern Resource for Healing
Enlighten Alternative Healing, LLC, 2013

Living Healthy & Happily Ever After
Rebecca Linder Hintze and Dr. Susan Lawton, 2012

Ayurveda & Aromatherapy – The Earth Essential Guide to Ancient Wisdom and Modern Healing
Dr. Light Miller, ND and Dr. Bryan Miller, DC, 1995

Aromatherapy for the Soul – Healing the Spirit with Fragrance and Essential Oils
Valerie Ann Worwood, 1999

Aromatherapy for Healing the Spirit – Restoring Emotion and Mental Balance with Essential Oils
Gabriel Mojay, 1997

The Aromatherapy Encyclopedia: A Concise Guide to Over 385 Plant Oils
Carol Schiller and David Schiller, 2008

The Directory of Essential Oils
Wanda Sellar, 1997

The Blossoming Heart – Aromatherapy for Healing and Transformation
Robbi Zeck, ND, 2008

The Fragrant Mind: Aromatherapy for Personality, Mind, Mood and Emotion
Valerie Ann Worwood, 1996

Resources and Supplies:

www.aromatools.com or **www.myoilbusiness.com** for Oil Display Racks,
Reference Guidebooks, Accessories, Class Tear Pads

www.shareoils.com for Informational Booklets

www.greenair.com for Diffusers

Appreciation for The EssentialYoga Program

*"I vividly remember my first dōTERRA essential oil yoga class with Jane at Downtown Desert Yoga! It was such a totally complete experience with dōTERRA oils – the room was infused with oil as we entered the yoga studio. As we began our centering, we each had oils added to our water to drink during our yoga practice – **grapefruit** that day! Jane explained each oil and its use as we used them in our practice. During our practice we massaged certain oils into our feet and special muscle groups, helping relax and deepen our work. We also had drops of oil put in our hands so we could breathe them in. Finally, ending our practice with the dōTERRA oils, each person was given a relaxing head massage. It was such a wonderful introduction to dōTERRA oils, the ways that they can be used, and how beautifully they enhance and deepen a yoga experience"*

    – JOANNA JONAS, LAS CRUCES, NM

"I teach an aromatherapy meditation program here in Germany. Although not yoga, our intention is to create a calming presence and help people get in better touch with themselves. Using the oils in meditation workshops creates a greater spiritual connection with more intense feelings of inner self or inner freedom. My students have told me they feel a more powerful connection or intensity in their practice using the oils, as well as a variation from meditation sessions without the oils. The oils help us to liberate the individual or open their awareness to new levels of understanding. My students are absolutely grateful for this new concept!"

    – MICHELLE TERNEDDE, BECHHOFEN, GERMANY

*"I never knew how enhanced my practice would be just by incorporating the sense of smell. Among many other benefits the oils have brought me, I particularly love that I could use **DigestZen** during the third trimester of my pregnancy for severe heartburn at night. I teach a class on Sunday nights that is slow-paced, candlelit and used to average 10-17 people a week. After incorporating the oils, I now get 30-40 people a week on average. Oil application doubles my class."*

    – DENISE GONZALES, ALBUQUERQUE, NM

"I assisted with a special dōTERRA essential oil yoga class on a few occasions, applying the oils throughout as the instructor guided the students through the practice that day. I find the essential oils help us to be more grounded and help intensify the power of yoga. Sharing the oils with the yoga students has helped our dōTERRA business grow. The people taking classes want to learn more about the therapeutic impact of the oils because they can feel immediately how effective the oils can be."

    – JOSET LOEWEN, BROOKS, ALBERTA, CANADA

"As an instructor and occupational therapist, I am always looking for a tool, a vehicle to help my students let go a little more, or to get to that next level. When introduced to dōTERRA oils during class, I realized I had found the medium to transform my teaching and others' practice...on so many levels."

    – KIM CHORMICLE, LAS CRUCES, NM

"I started sharing the oils because I love them so much. My enthusiasm and authentic love for the dōTERRA essential oils has encouraged others to use the oils with great success. I have not been sick for over 1 1/2 years since I started using the oils. As a yoga teacher, dōTERRA essential oils have provided opportunities for me to teach unique classes and workshops that expand consciousness of mind, body and spirit. My students love being touched with the oils."

    – LISA KNELLER, SCOTTSDALE, AZ

"I've noticed that using the oils has allowed me to release judgment about where I am in my practice. I feel as though I am more present in each moment and able to harness the benefits both yoga and essential oils offer. The combination of yoga and daily oil use has allowed me to stay healthy and has given me energy...I love that! As a Reiki practitioner, I love incorporating the oils. They have served as effective tools allowing my clients to relax deeper and heal faster. I can't wait to use them in designing my own yoga classes – the theme possibilities are endless! I have found the essential oil yoga classes are a great way to offer potential oil users an experience. In the grand scheme of things, this is probably what has benefited my dōTERRA business the most."

    – NICOLE HARINGS, LAS CRUCES, NM

"Using dōTERRA essential oils in my classes gives me ideas for themes and postures. When I am preparing to teach I sit and think about what I want to bring into the class that day. Sometimes I select the oil ahead of time and the class flows from there. For instance, I might want to use **geranium** *and since I know it is good for heart opening, I lead a class that opens the heart. Teaching essential oil yoga classes gives me the opportunity to share dōTERRA with my students in a fun and creative way. Many of the students LOVE particular oils and end up purchasing them. Students often come to the dōTERRA classes that I teach and bring their friends. The oils give me a nice way to introduce the oils and invite students to classes."*

    – ROSE KRESS, TUCSON, AZ

"The essential oils have helped me by allowing me to stop the mind chatter and really be focused and present during my yoga practice. I feel that my allergies have been minimized and lung capacity increased as I breathe deeper and focus on my breathing more when using the essential oils in my practice. You have to experience the oils to really appreciate their power and benefits, otherwise you won't believe what others tell you."

    – NORMA WONG-SULPEVEDA, EL PASO, TX

"I use dōTERRA essential oils as an integral part of my yoga practice. It helps me drop out of my thoughts and create an effect in my practice. I often use **frankincense** *at the third eye as part of my meditation practice. Using the essential oils has added a value of experience to my students' practice as well. My students often ask me, "Did you bring any oils today?" It has become a special part of the class for them. Since I've been using the essential oils, I've bought less over-the-counter medicine and cleaning products. dōTERRA essential oils are my first choice for my home and health care. I feel confident using them and sharing such high-quality products."*

    – SHANEE WOLF, CAVE CREEK, AZ

About Us

The EssentialYoga Program was developed in collaboration with the four of us below. Each brings our own unique experiences and perspective on essential oils and yoga. We enthusiastically present dōTERRA® essential oils in this Program to the greater yoga community as another powerful dimension to enhance the practice, teachings and business of yoga.

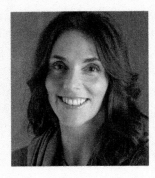

Jane Bloom

jane@essentialyogaprogram.com

Jane Bloom lives in beautiful Mesilla, New Mexico with her husband and three boys. She enjoys holding a space for others to deepen their self-awareness and growth. Jane earned her master's degree in Counseling Educational Psychology and has practiced as a family therapist for the past 12 years. She specializes in group counseling, pioneering one of the first postpartum support groups in New Mexico and working with families of children with autism. She has practiced yoga for the past 20 years and is a certified yoga instructor. She teaches a variety of yoga classes, including hot, vinyasa flow and gentle yoga in an accessible way. She enjoys teaching yoga to children and specializes in Parent & Baby Yoga with a focus on attachment and social emotional development.

dōTERRA essential oils fit into every aspect of Jane's life. She was immediately taken with how the oils afford her family holistic healthcare. The oils were a natural fit with her love of counseling, where she has integrated them into her work with children and families. Combining her background in counseling and yoga, Jane is particularly interested in how creative sequencing with oils elicits emotions and changes awareness one asana at a time. Jane is excited to share the integration of essential oils and yoga, which have the common goal of helping others find balance in their lives.

dōTERRA essential oils provide endless creativity in teaching yoga, and continually inspire monthly EssentialYoga workshops that students are drawn to for a powerful restorative and cathartic experience. Jane has enjoyed hosting EssentialYoga workshops around the country, in addition to offering instructor trainings with the oils. As the essential oils inspire, Jane invites her students to explore their practice with an open heart and mind. She is grateful for her family and contributions from her many instructors along this journey, including the mentorship and support of her amazing dōTERRA team.

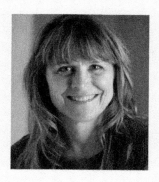

Marty Harger
marty@essentialyogaprogram.com

Marty Harger was introduced to yoga while attending freestyle ski camp in Wyoming in the late 1970s – her first trip to the western USA. Her introduction to essential oils came a few years later as did her increasing awareness of the body's powerful ability to heal itself with natural approaches. In midlife, Marty hopped off the big-city corporate fast-track and began her personal and professional journey to find her niche in the healing arts. It was during that year of massage school in Chicago that her passion for essential oils really took hold. What began with aromatherapy studies evolved into the use of therapeutic grade essential oils as she was introduced to dōTERRA in 2008 at the wellness center she owns in the mountains of Heber City, Utah. A ski bum at heart, Marty and her husband moved back to Utah in 2003 to live in a setting that inspired them where she opened her own practice, Balance – Therapeutic Massage and Wellness Center. She is active in her community, serving in leadership roles for the local chamber of commerce/convention bureau, as well as co-founding a health and wellness practitioners networking group.

Marty feels she has found her niche in the world of natural health practices as a nationally certified massage therapist since 2000, and in recent years, becoming a certified instructor in dōTERRA's essential oil-based **AromaTouch Technique.** Marty adores working with her international dōTERRA team of Wellness Advocates to help teach others about the benefits and healing power of essential oils. She feels honored to lead such a successful group of entrepreneurs to reach their life dreams through the dōTERRA businesses they are building.

She is a born "connector" of people and has always loved the process of creating and launching new ventures. Marty finds dōTERRA a great match with endless ways to learn, do and teach others. She feels strongly about the importance of what The EssentialYoga Program offers. She is a yoga student who enjoys taking classes wherever she can in her hometown and when she travels. She finds great fun in co-teaching EssentialYoga, working with her dōTERRA teammates to apply the oils with yoga instructor friends. Marty finds the essential oils are a source of continued inspiration for future endeavors! She absolutely LOVES her life in the mountains of Utah, the fabulous new friends she's met through her years with dōTERRA, and the financial support and choices it affords her every day to live a life others dream about! She is so very grateful.

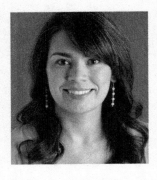

Deidra Schaub

deidra@essentialyogaprogram.com

Deidra Schaub is a restorative yoga instructor specializing in yin yoga since 2012. She is originally from northern New Mexico, where she grew up experiencing creativity through her artist father, and alternative healing through her mother, who practices Healing Touch. As a home-schooling mom, Deidra uses dōTERRA essential oils for cleaning, cooking and as the medicine of choice for her family. She particularly enjoys using the essential oils to craft her own natural skin care products, such as lotions, body washes and scrubs. She now lives in southern New Mexico where she has carved out a unique niche.

Deidra has a passion for supporting and volunteering for social justice and environmental awareness causes in her community. That passion, along with her love of art, led to creating jewelry with repurposed papers. She loves working alongside other artists as a member of a creative cooperative. She displays her work in various art shows, galleries and an environmental center in New Mexico. She even has found a way to combine three unlikely passions: teaching Yoga & Creativity Workshops, where students experience the powerful combination of essential oils and yoga to tap in to creative intelligence, and co-teaching live music yoga sessions with Jane Bloom, where students experience spontaneous aromatherapy yoga sequencing to musical improvisation.

Deidra has been practicing yoga for several years and has found the combination of oils and yoga effective to assist her in managing anxiety and depression while deepening her connection to God and her Christian faith. She decided to become an instructor after attending a 200-hour yoga instructor training to expand her own practice. She soon discovered her gift for teaching those who are intimidated by the traditional image of yoga or view yoga as nothing more than exercise. Deidra brings a sense of balance and accessibility to how instructors can share the concepts presented in The EssentialYoga Program, helping us make sure there are options for all levels. It is her goal to make sure we "leave no one behind" in our approach to using oils in yoga.

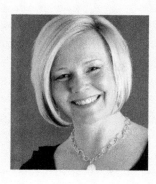

Stephanie Smith

stephanie@essentialyogaprogram.com

Stephanie Smith's path from the dance studio to the yoga studio began when she was a young girl exploring ballet, jazz and tap. After a few years as a college dance major, she left her home state of Utah for a professional dance career in Los Angeles. That road led to ventures in personal training and fitness as well as teaching dance to others since 1984. Her love of yoga began in 1996 as she explored Bikram, or hot yoga. Ever curious, Stephanie continued her yoga instructor training in many forms over the years and a growing interest in the mind-body connection. Her unique style brings a sense of curiosity and inquiry into the studio as she meets yoga students where they are and helps guide them to a deeper understanding of their body, mind and spirit.

Stephanie is a certified yoga instructor with over 500 hours of accredited instructor trainings, including Ashtanga, Anusara, Iveyngar, Viniyoga and yoga therapeutics. Her essential oil experience began years ago as she introduced aromatherapy into her yoga classes on a regular basis. She considers herself "forever a student," but also feels it is her life's calling to magnify the skills of other instructors. Stephanie often travels around the country to conduct yoga instructor training programs that incorporate essential oils. She is especially grateful to all of her instructors and colleagues who have enabled her to be who she is today.

Stephanie has the heart of an entrepreneur, which is evident in her life path. She has taken the lead as dance studio owner, as an independent yoga instructor in Scottsdale, Arizona studios, and more recently with a thriving dōTERRA essential oils business. She often focuses her work in therapeutic yoga, including private lessons, social gatherings and private and group instructor trainings. Recently Stephanie and her family moved back to Utah, where she has helped establish a thriving yoga community in a small mountain town. She is excited to offer this blend of yoga and oils that bring together some of her learnings over 17 years creating classes that have touched hundreds of lives.

Endnotes

1

World Health Organization article: www.who.int/bulletin/volumes/86/8/07-042820/en

2

Web MD.com article: www.webmd.com/balance/guide/ayurvedic-treatments

3

University of Nebraska article: http://dwb.unl.edu/teacher/nsf/C10/C10Links/ericir.syr.edu/Projects/
Newton/11/tstesmll

4, 21, 22, 23, 29, 33, 37, 38, 39, 42, 43, 45, 61, 63, 66
Modern Essentials – A Contemporary Guide to the Therapeutic Use of Essential Oils
AromaTools, 2013

5, 6, 7, 8, 9, 10, 11, 12, 14, 15, 17, 19, 20, 27, 30, 31, 34, 35, 36, 44, 46, 47, 49, 51, 52, 53, 54, 57, 58,
62, 64, 65
Emotions & Essential Oils – A Modern Resource for Healing
Enlighten Alternative Healing, LLC, 2012

13, 48, 55
The Blossoming Heart – Aromatherapy for Healing and Transformation
Robbi Zeck, ND, 2008

16, 18, 32, 40, 41
Aromatherapy for the Soul – Healing the Spirit with Fragrance and Essential Oils
Valerie Ann Worwood, 1999

24, 25, 26, 28
The Fragrant Mind – Aromatherapy for Personality, Mind, Mood and Emotion
Valerie Ann Worwood, 1996

56
Aromatherapy for Healing the Spirit – Restoring Emotional and Mental Balance with Essential Oils
Gabriel Mojay, 1997

59, 60
Living Healthy & Happily Ever After
Rebecca Linder Hintze and Dr. Susan Lawton, 2012

67
Pricing effective March 1, 2014 as listed by dōTERRA International, LLC. for U.S. wholesale
product prices

CPSIA information can be obtained at www.ICGtesting.com
Printed in the USA
LVOW05s0731300415

436534LV00008BA/21/P